I0435337

Cancer Cure Success Guide©
Proven Ways to Treat, Cure and Prevent Cancer and Other Chronic Illnesses

Written by Sage Crystal

Table of Contents

About the Author

Sage Crystal, a native Philadelphian, who excelled in athletics and achieved many accolades and awards stemming back to her days of youth athletics. She continued on the athletic path throughout adulthood. Sage thrived in the field of fitness becoming a bodybuilder and personal trainer while also owning a catering business that centered on wholesome, gourmet style cuisine.

She took her passion for sports performance and wholesome nutrition to new levels in her coaching and teaching methods. Sage helps others from their starting line by empowering and mentoring them to embark on a life changing journey into healthy living.

As a well sought after fitness trainer in the Philadelphia area, she specializes in holistic exercise, functional movement, and other diverse fitness modalities. Learning from personal family experiences, Sage uses her expertise as a certified nutrition specialist and taps her expertise in Neurolinguistic Programming (NLP), to teach and inform others, to help overcome illness, lose weight, raise their level of health and wellbeing, to improve all aspects of their lives, which also includes helping them to understand and live a spiritual-centered lifestyle.

For over ten years, Sage has immersed herself in the alternative health field and is currently studying to become a Naturopathic Doctor. She has widely read and intensely researched for the best resources in natural and alternative health.

Sage is a Certified Life Coach, co-founder and member of *The Core of 8: Integrated Coaching Network,* whose vision is to provide the most advanced coaching services to help clients improve their lifestyles and wellbeing, by helping them set specific goals, making a plan of action and following it to reach desired outcomes.

In addition to her work in life coaching, fitness and nutrition, Sage is also a professional writer and has authored numerous books and articles in the fields of natural health, fitness, and spirituality. Sage can be reached via her email address: Sage@SageCrystal.net

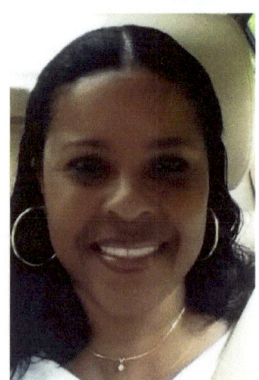

Introduction

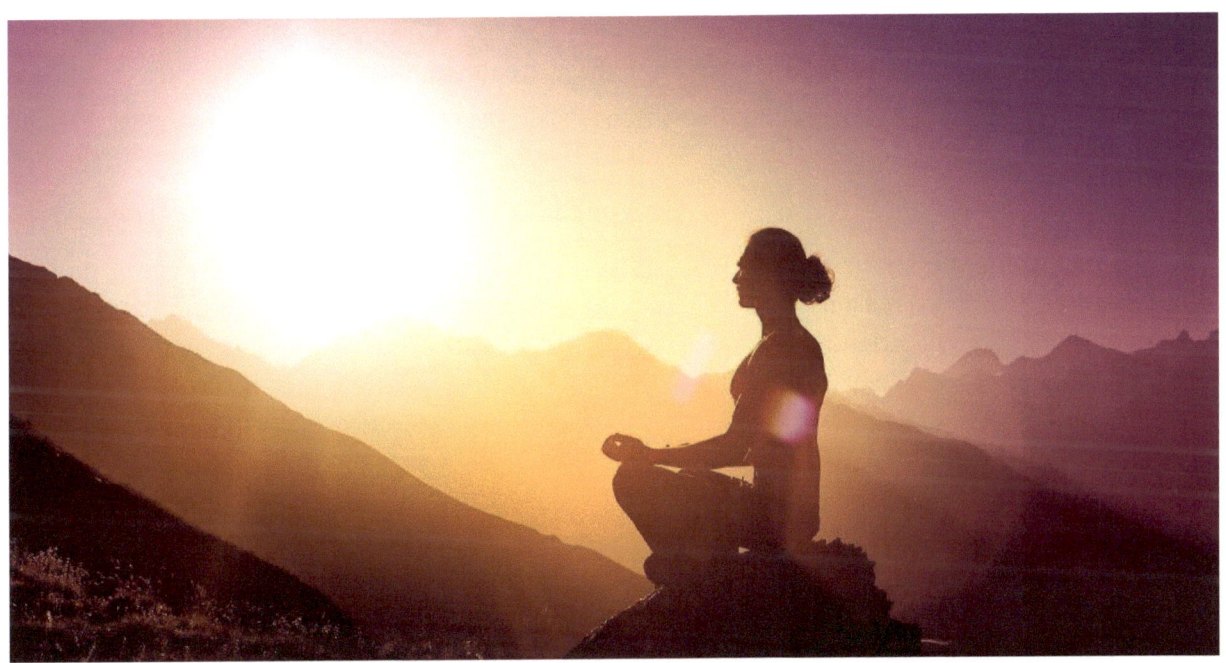

Cancer is big business. The average treatment per patient is over $50,000, yet the mortality rates are staggering. The success record of today's cancer doctors with their zealous "kill-or-cure" approach is dismal. They achieve remission in about 7% of cancer patients. In an additional 15% of cases, the life of the patient is marginally prolonged. They call it a "cure" if the patient hangs on for 5 years, even if he dies a day later. This miserable track record of a chemical assault, so brutal and morbid, for many patients, the mere thought of having another chemo or radiation treatment can trigger the vomit reflex.

Many patients develop "chemo-brain," a decline of memory and other cognitive functions. Chemotherapy lowers the body's oxygen level (cancer cells thrive in a low-oxygen environment) and interjects an extremely poisonous substance into the body that kills much more than cancer cells. It further ravages an immune system that is severely compromised already. A virtually collapsed immune system makes chemo-radiation cancer patients easy prey to all types of other diseases. Many patients are unable to digest food after these treatments because the friendly flora and bacteria within the system have been killed-off, and patients starve to death before the cancer can kill them.

The National Cancer Institute reported that up to 40% of cancer patients die of malnutrition or other diseases. For these reasons, chemotherapy or radiation is usually the "kiss of death." Well-meaning, but ignorant friends or relatives often pressure cancer patients into going for conventional treatments, which they later too often regret. Too many only go to alternative therap/y after conventional therapy has worsened their condition and done extensive, often irreparable damage.

Former talk show host and White House Press Secretary, Tony Snow was diagnosed with colon cancer 3 years before he died. Even after 6 months of chemotherapy and the removal of the colon – to be on the "safe" side as it was called – the cancer spread to the liver, leading to his demise. Tony was an intelligent guy, but fatally naïve when it came to choosing proper treatments for his illness.

Farrah Fawcett had extensive chemotherapy and radiation. After 6 months, she was declared "cancer free" – and after another 6 months, she died. President Ronald Reagan was wise enough to avoid lethal American cancer treatments. In 1985 he had his colon cancer cured by Ozone specialist Dr. Hans Nieper in Hannover, Germany. Dr. Nieper later commented: "You wouldn't believe how many FDA officials or their relatives and directors of the AMA and other American cancer associations come to see me as patients in Hannover. Strange, that the same therapies they deny people in their own country are good enough for them abroad."

A recent survey of the 64 staff members at the McGill Cancer Therapy Center in Montreal revealed that 58 or 90% would reject chemotherapy for themselves or their family. It is also known that health care workers who came in direct contact with chemotherapy substances have contracted cancer. The American Cancer Society reports that, "Some 550,000 cancer patients die each year in the U.S., primarily from chemotherapy."

Dr. Robert Atkins whose name has become a household word since his book on a low carbohydrate diet, said: "There is not one, but many cures for cancer. But they are all being systematically suppressed by the American Cancer Society, The National Cancer Institute, the AMA, the FDA, and the major oncology centers. They have too much of a vested interest in the status quo." For example, Dr. William Frederick Koch's revolutionary Glyoxylide therapy was railroaded because it worked too well. Acclaimed health authority Dr. John Heinerman wrote that in tests done at Sloan Kettering, Laetrile had a definite inhibitory effect on lung cancer, but officials at Sloan Kettering informed the press that all tests with Laetrile turned out to be negative. After analyzing cancer statistics for several decades of patients treated with orthodox therapies, Dr. Hardin Jones, a professor at the University of California with 25 years of experience, concluded: Patients are as well or better off, untreated. My studies have proven conclusively those cancer patients who refuse chemotherapy and radiation actually live up to four times longer that treated cases, including untreated Breast Cancer cases."

Cancer Physician, Dr. Charles Moerthel of the Mayo Clinic, stated: "Our most effective regiments are fraught with risks and side-effects and practical problems; and after this price is paid by all the patients we have treated, only a small fraction are rewarded with a transient period of usually tumor regression." Dr. Samuel Epstein put into the Congressional Record in1987: "Chemotherapy and radiation can increase the risk of developing a second cancer by up to 100 times." Dr. Otis Brawley, chief medical officer of the American Cancer Society disclosed: "It is ironic but true that many cancer chemotherapies are known to cause (a secondary) cancer." Dr. Kenneth Forror adds: "I'm the patient now and I don't have to follow that (chemo) routine. It never did that much good. I had to keep prescribing it to keep my hospital privileges." Albert Braverman, M.D. wrote an article that was published in the Lancet, in which he stated: "Most cancer patients in this country die of chemotherapy. Chemotherapy does not eliminate breast, colon or lung cancers, yet doctors still use chemotherapy for these tumors."

Italian oncologist and author, Tulio Simoncini, M.D. says that an overgrowth of candida albicans facilitates cancer and points out that chemotherapy lays the groundwork for candida proliferation. Chemotherapy expert Ernst Wynder, a former professor at Sloan-Kettering Hospital, wrote this warning to professor Michael Gearing-Tosh about advising a close friend regarding chemotherapy: "If your friend touches chemotherapy, he's a goner." Dr. Richard E. Eby, Obstetrician, professor and author, once approached the AMA and asked why no serious studies were ever made of primitive societies where the people have no cancer, whereas cancer was so prevalent in America. Being a famous doctor and medical leader, the AMA could not ignore him. They therefore referred him to their chief counsel. He asked Dr. Eby if he had ever read the bylaws of the AMA. He then explained that the main purpose of the AMA was to protect the income of its members.   Therefore the AMA would make sure that no cancer cure was ever found or recognized in this country. End of discussion! Not stated but understood was that carefully placed political "contributions" (pronounced – Bribes) to members of Congress would insure that the FDA carried out the AMA policy! Many courageous physicians who have used "unapproved" innovative natural therapies have been railroaded, put out of business and even thrown into jail.

This book will bring you **190 effective natural cancer therapies**, some of them old and some brand new. You will be amazed at the simple and inexpensive remedies that have been available to anybody who looks for them. Father Romano Zalgado from the Belem Monastery in Portugal has been helping cancer patients with his natural remedy for decades. Nobel nominee, Dr. Budwig, has discovered an inexpensive and effective remedy that works especially well for prostate cancer. How about the remedy made from a Native American tree that isolates cancer cells and cuts off their blood supply causing them to die. Or how about the alternative doctor who has cured over 40,000 cancer patients with a special raw vegetable juice regiment? Do you think chemo-doctors would tell you about any of these natural remedies? Due to ignorance or conflict of interest they may rather let you die than to direct you to anything that is above and beyond orthodox quackery. Conventional cancer treatments would make the critical analyst laugh if it wasn't so serious. Soon, Cancer Surgery, Radiation and Chemotherapy will be looked upon as erroneous procedures that were practiced in the "dark ages" of medicine.

Discover treatments that have worked miracles for many, designed by naturopathic doctors who have turned doomed cancer victims into elated survivors. The side effects of these remedies will not kill you – because there aren't any. The book also refers to consultation, referral, and treatment centers.

I.   One Hundred and Ninety Natural Cancer Therapies

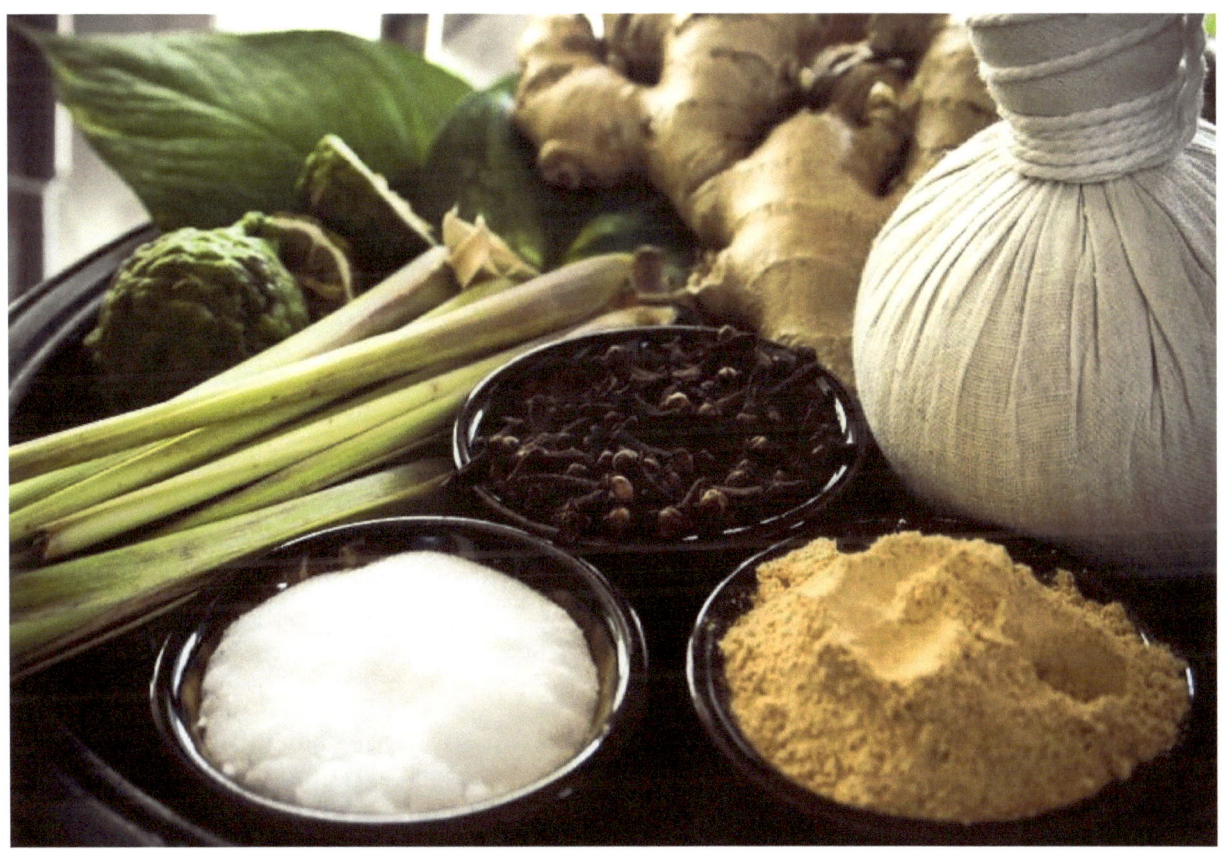

In her book *"The Cure for all Cancers,"* researcher Dr. Hulda Clark maintains that all cancers are caused by a parasite (fluke). This parasite lives in the intestine where it does little harm. It is only when it invades other organs that it causes serious diseases, including cancer/ According to the author, the herbs when taken together, can rid the body of virtually all types of parasites, enabling the body to defeat the cancer. After ingesting the remedy for about a week, the fluke in all its stages is eradicated. The book is available in most stores. Alternatively, you can order it from New Century Press for about $16 at 800-519-2465 or 317-666-8741.

1. Maitake

Numerous studies and tests have shown that the Chinese medicinal mushroom, **Maitake**, has definite anti-cancer and anti-tumor properties. Some of the patients successfully treated with Maitake were suffering from prostate and brain cancer. Although Maitake may not necessarily bring about a complete cure, it almost always improves the patient's condition considerably. The Maitake product generally recommended is Grifron-Pro D-Fraction. For therapeutic effects a daily dosage of 35 to 70 drops is recommended. The product is available from: Maitake Products at: 800-747-7418.

2. Licorice Root

According to health experts, simple **licorice root** is a dynamic disease beater that can defeat cancer and even conquer AIDS. Research has shown that Phytochemicals (or plant vitamins) have amazing powers to boost the immune system, and this miraculous root is full of them. They are extremely effective in combating the growth and development of cancer cells, especially prostate and breast cancer cells. Herbal licorice products are available in most Health Food stores.

3. Breast Milk

According to Swedish research, **breast milk** contains a substance that kills cancer cells. A compound called A-lactalbumin (MAL) triggers a process called apoptosis, or cell suicide, in cancer cells but not in normal cells. In one experiment, 98% of all human lung cancer cells were killed. According to the report, the milk compound also induced apoptosis in cancer cells in the kidney, bladder and intestines.

4. Essiac

Rene Caisse was in possession of an old Indian cancer remedy. During the 1920s and 30s, she was busy curing cancer patients. Her services were always free of charge and she lived only on voluntary donations. To the chagrin of the medical and drug establishment she became famous as a successful healer. She was constantly harassed and arrested many times for "practicing medicine without license". She also resisted many attempts to sell out her secret formula, knowing it would be kept from the people, or used to make huge profits for the pharmaceutical industry. At her funeral in the Canadian village of Bracebridge (north of Toronto), hundreds of former cancer patients paid their last respects to the woman who had so selflessly saved their lives. **Essiac** is Rene's last name spelled backwards. For more information, do a web search for "Essiac Handbook".

5. Father Romano Zalgado's Cancer Remedy

Ingredients:

- 2 lbs. of unheated and unfiltered raw honey
- 2 large or 3 small leaves of Aloe Vera
- 3 or 4 soupspoons of whisky or brandy

Directions:

Clean the Aloe Vera and remove the thorns. Cut into small pieces. Put all ingredients into a blender and liquefy. Take one soupspoon 15 minutes before each meal. This amount should last you for at least 10 days.

6. Cat's Claw

This South American herb has traditionally helped many desperately ill cancer patients. **Cat's Claw** of the most potent quality is available from Carotec at: 800-522-4279.

7. Evening Primrose Oil

According to reports by the South African Medical Journal, research indicated that gammalinolenic acid taken from **evening primrose oil** kills human cancer cells, and without side effects. Cancer cells multiply when the immune system is weak. Evening primrose oil may help by converting into PGE1, which has a crucial effect on the immune system, stimulating the T-Cells and keeping the cell membranes healthy. Although no conclusive information is available yet, the Bristol Cancer Help Center (England) is recommending evening primrose oil as one of the nutritional therapies. It's available in most Health Food stores.

8. Gerson Therapy

One widely known and successful alternative treatment is administered to the directions of a German doctor, whose therapy is based on a strict, regimented organic diet. The **Gerson Therapy** offers patients with cancer, AIDS and other so-called incurable diseases an excellent chance of winning the fight against cancer. For details, call: 619-685-5353 or 888-4-GERSON.

9. Cancer Control Society

The **Cancer Control Society** offers educational material in the prevention and cure of cancer and other nutrition related diseases. Information on non-toxic therapies and doctors is available at a nominal charge. For details, call: 323-663-7801

10. Organic Germanium

The National Cancer Institute has accepted organic germanium as a therapeutic approach in the treatment of cancer and AIDS. Organic germanium's health benefits go beyond simply increasing available oxygen which by itself is detrimental to cancer cells. It also appears to be a powerful immune enhancer. Studies are supported by hundreds of clinical studies in which organic germanium cured "incurable" diseases. No negative side effects were observed. For product information contact:

- I-Herb at: 323-663-7801
- Bio Institute at: 800-866-6786

11. Rebounding

Bouncing on a small (or big) trampoline from 10-30 minutes daily has definite health benefits for the sick as well as the healthy. The temporary suspension of gravity is a universal cell exercise which enhances cell communication. The healthy cells "persuade" the cancerous cells to return to normal. This is a proven alternative method to fight cancer. To be used to compliment other natural approaches. Recommended reading: *"The Cancer Answer,"* by Albert Earl Cater. Available in book stores or from Medak Mfg. at: 800-232-5762.

12. The Budwig Diet

Researcher Dr. Johanna Budwig found that the blood of cancer patients is deficient or void of the fatty acids Albumin and Ester Phosphatide, which are crucial for normal cell division. Dr. Budwig discovered that a combination of approximately 1 tbsp. or organic cold-pressed flax seed oil mixed with 1 heaping tbsp. of low fat cottage cheese (ration of about 1 to 2) restores the blood to its normal condition and oxygenates the cells. Within a period of about 3-4 months, tumors gradually recede, and the symptoms of cancer are often totally eliminated. The remedy is taken daily, preferably a half hour before breakfast. This food combination has also been shown to be beneficial for arteriosclerosis, liver dysfunction, arthritis, diabetes, eczema, bronchial spasms and irregular heartbeat. The formula is most effective if mixed in a blender. Organic cold-pressed flax seed oil and organic low fat cottage cheese are both available in most health food stores. Other flavor enhancing natural ingredients may be added after mixing. Recommended reading: *"How to Fight Cancer and Win,"* by William L. Fisher.

13. Graviola

Extract from this South American tree selectively targets and kills malignant cells in 12 types of Cancer, including colon, breast, prostate, lung and pancreatic cancer. Since 1976 **graviola** has been proven to be and immensely potent cancer killer in 20 independent laboratory tests, yet it as never become part of any mainstream cancer protocol. For more information:

- Visit: www.rain-forest.com

Graviola is available from:

- Amazon Herb Company at: 800-835-0850
- Raintree Nutrition at: 800-780-5902

14. Laetrile Sources

Laetrile is not available in the U.S., but it can be legally bought overseas for personal use. It is usually used in conjunction with other natural therapies. For product information, do a quick web search or call:

- 800-291-1508
- 800-851-9470

15. Paw-Paw

Paw-Paw is a North American tree of the custard-apple family, with purple flowers and a yellow edible fruit. When ingested, it isolates cancer cells by cutting off their blood supply, causing them to die. Tests have shown that tumors, including lung and brain, reduce in size and usually vanish completely. A very effective cancer treatment. For product information, do quick web searches for "Paw-Paw against cancer" or call:

- Nature Sunshine at: 888-523-1727
- New Beginnings in Health at: 877-871-6262

16. Alternative Medicine: Definitive Guide to Cancer

This 1,120 page book illustrated many successful alternative approaches that can remove the root causes of cancer and restore your health without further weakening or poisoning your body. Over 30 top physicians explain their successful alternative treatments. The guide is available for approximately $50 in book stores (ISBN# 1887299017).

17. Fluoride and Refined Sugar

If you are afflicted with cancer (or wish to prevent it), it is indispensable that you **refrain from fluoridated water and refined white sugar**. Japanese scientists have proven that the same levels of fluoride commonly put into U.S. water supplies are capable of transforming normal cells into cancer cells. Research sponsored in 1963 by the American Cancer Institute clearly showed that even very low levels of fluoride increased the incidence of tumors in experimental animals by a frightening 12% to 100%. Research also showed that common refined sugar is linked to cancer. Cancer cells thrive in a sugar-rich environment. Sugar consumed in fresh fruit does not have the same effect.

18. User Forum

Therapy feed-back from cancer patients:

- www.datehookup.com/Thread-96135.htm

19. Noni Juice

- The juice of the Polynesian fruit has been used for centuries to cure virtually any disease, including cancer. For more information, do a quick web search or call:
- Whole Health at: 800-382-1936
- NJP Products at: 800-657-7763
- Noni Connection at: 888-335-6664

20. The Atkins Center

Located in New York City, this hospital uses a variety of natural therapies, supported by an appropriate diet. Telephone consultations are also available. For more information, call: 800-ATKINS-8.

21. Hydrazine Sulfate

Hydrazine sulfate has been used for 25 years by thousands of desperate cancer patients with excellent results. This non-toxic drug is an inexpensive cancer fighter. It works by depriving cancer cells from the nourishment they need to proliferate. It also seems to have conciliatory effects when taken during chemotherapy, and especially during radiation treatment. However, it is not compatible with alcohol, tranquilizers, sedatives, anti-depressants or anti-anxiety drugs. Because this supplement is relatively inexpensive and effective, it is relentlessly suppressed by the cancer merchants. Kathy Keeton, the wife of Penthouse publisher Bob Guccione, recovered from terminal metastatic breast cancer, which has spread to various other parts of her body. The most commonly recommended dosage is one 60mg capsule before breakfast on days 1 to 3, one 60mg capsule before breakfast and one 60mg capsule before dinner on days 4 to 6, one 60mg capsule before breakfast, one 60mg capsule before dinner and one 60mg capsule before the last meal before bedtime thereafter. For product information do a quick web search or contact:

- American Health Alternatives at: 406-543-2912
- Nu-gen Nitrogen at: 800-446-8184
- National Cancer Institute at: 800-422-6237
- Life Energy Distributors at: 604-856-0171

22. Zyflamend

This product is comprised of 10 specific herbs. It has shown the ability to decrease COX-2 activity as well as potent toxic drugs. Prostate cancer cell proliferation was reduced by up to 75%. For more information, call:

I-Herb at: 951-616-3600
Health Fair at: 800-366-6056

23. Photoluminescence

This therapy modulates the immune response by changing the antigenic structure in blood cells. The procedure intravenously exposes some of the blood to strong ultraviolet light. The modulation can last up to 40 weeks after treatment. The therapy has shown to be of great benefit in the fight against cancer as well as many other diseases. For more information call Health Sciences Institute at: 800-981-7157. For nationwide clinics, visit: www.cancure.org/directory_clinics.htm.

24. Herbal Teas

There are around a hundred different types of cancer. The following herbs have been used for generations by folk healers to prevent and treat cancer: red clover, black radish, dandelion, Pau D'Acro (purple LaPacho), sorrel, fenugreek, rosemary. Get some of them from your local health food store, mix them and make teas. Drink on a regular basis instead of coffee.

25. Late Stage Prostate Cancer

For referrals to local doctors experienced in using combined hormone blockade, cryo-ablation therapy, seed implantation and more, call PAACT at: 616-453-1477. There is no charge for this service, but small donations are appreciated.

26. Hoxsey Bio-Medical Center

Harry Hoxsey, at the age of 18, founded the Hoxsey Cancer Clinic in Dallas in 1919. He used the herbal formulas developed by his veterinarian great-grandfather. By the 1950s, the Hoxsey Cancer Clinic had become one of the largest privately-owned medical facilities in the world. Unfortunately, years of harassment by the FDA and AMA pressured him to close his clinic. He gave his head nurse, Mildred Nelson, his formulas and in 1963 she established the **Bio-Medical Center** in Tijuana. The cornerstone of the Hoxsey therapy is the Hoxsey herbal tonics. The formulas include bloodroot, burdock, buckthorn, cascara, barberry, licorice, red clover, pokeroot, zinc chloride and antimony tri-sulfate. In addition to the herbal tonics, Mildred Nelson added a special diet to the treatment, which does not allow the consumption of pork, vinegar, tomatoes, pickles, carbonated drinks, alcohol, bleached flour, sugar and most salts. The Hoxsey therapy also places great importance on a positive mental attitude by the patient. Unlike other clinics, treatment is more flexible here. Patients are often treated on an out-patient basis. After determining the patient's needs, they may return home with a three-month supply of tonics. There is a $3,500 flat fee for a lifetime supply of tonics. In addition, there is a nominal charge for various services such as diagnosis, x-rays, lab tests and so forth. Mildred Nelson claims that approximately 80% of the patients are helped at varying degrees. Many patients are hard-core that they were given up for dead by conventional doctors. For more information, contact the Bio-Medical Center. Address:

- P.O. Box 433654
  San Ysidor, CA 92143-3654
- Tel: 011-52-644-684-90-11 (Mexico)

27. Oasis of Hope

This treatment center was founded by the pioneer of Mexico's alternative therapists, Dr. Ernesto Contreras, over 35 years ago. The therapy is custom tailored for each cancer patients. Aspects of the metabolic program include: laetrile, shark cartilage, correct nutrition, detoxification, chelation and ozone therapy. Emotional and spiritual issues are also addressed. The hospital has had the best success rate with prostate cancer, breast cancer, colon cancer and lung cancer. Approximately 85% of patients experience a cure or improvement in their condition. For more information, call: Contreras Oasis of Hope at: 619-690-8450

28. Private Cancer Clinic Tours

You can get an impression; ask questions; and more by participating in a tour to the alternative cancer clinics in Tijuana and other Mexican cities at a reasonable rate. For more information, call:

- CCS Cancer Clinic Tours at: 209-529-4697
- Cancer Control Society at: 209-529-4697
- Or check out the following website: www.cancure.org/directory_mexican_clinics.htm

29. Multiple Therapies

Since all alternative cancer treatments have a different effect on different individuals, not every single cancer therapy may have the desired effect. Therefore, it is suggested to **use several therapies simultaneously**. Natural supplements and therapies – contrary to drugs – do not cause toxic interactions.

30. Healing Choices

Ralph W. Moss, Ph. D. is an advisor on alternate cancer treatment for the National Institute of Health, Columbia University, and the University of Texas. He researches and writes individual **Healing Choice** reports for people with Cancer. For details:

- Call: 800-980-1234.

- Visit: www.cancerdecisions.com

31. Ukrain

Ukrain is a plant alkaloid, and one of the most promising natural substances to fight cancer. Significant improvement often occurs within 2-4 weeks. Dr. Atkins regarded Ukrain as the single best anticancer agent he's ever used. Effective against most cancers. Ukrain is one of the therapies used at the Atkins Center in New York.

32. Broccoli

Broccoli, cauliflower and other cruciferous vegetables help protect against breast cancer. One of their ingredients, indole-3-carbinol, breaks estrogen down into inactive byproducts. Estrogen's active byproducts have been found to promote tumors. These vegetables are most effective if uncooked or lightly steamed, and organic.

33. People Against Cancer

This counseling service will evaluate each individual case and recommend the most appropriate alternative therapies. Their doctors travel far and wide to familiarize themselves with the latest proven treatments. For details call: 515-972-4444.

34. Whey

Tests have shown that animals fed **whey protein** before subjected to cancer causing agents, mounted a much more vigorous immune response than animals fed other types of protein. Whey has been found to deplete the glutathione level in cancer cells, without effecting healthy cells. Glutathione is a cellular oxygen carrier. Most whey products are processed in a manner that destroys most of the protein's ability to deplete cancer cells of glutathione. One of the most effective whey products is available from:

- www.DefenseNutrition.com

35. Bindweed

The extract of this plant effectively inhibits the growth of blood vessels to cancer cells. It is 100 times more effective than shark cartilage. For more details, contact:

- Oregon Wholistic Health Clinic at: 503-657-4043
- Aidan Products (Aidan's product is called C-Statin) at: 877-272-3508

36. Green Tea

A powerful antioxidant called "epigallo-catechin-3-gallatge" killed cancer cells in samples of skin, lymph system and prostate tissues taken from both humans and mice, while leaving healthy tissues unharmed. The tests were done by researchers from Case Western Reserve University in Cleveland, Ohio. A cup of **green tea** contains between 100 and 200mg of the anti-cancer ingredient. If used as therapy, a minimum of 4 cups should be consumed daily. May be combined with rosemary tea for enhanced effect.

37. MGN-3

This natural, non-toxic product is one of the most powerful immune boosters. It is a combination of extracts of rice bran and the mushrooms Shiitake, Kawaratake and Suehirotake. **MGN-3** works well for all types of cancers, including multiple myeloma, viral hepatitis B and C and leukemia. Treatment has been beneficial to AIDS patients as well. Tests have shown a 60-70% decrease in cancer cells after just 2 weeks in 99% of patients. For product information call:
* CompassioNet at: 800-510-2010
* Aloha Medicinals at: 877-835-6091

38. Visualization Therapy

According to many scientists, disease begins in the mind before in manifests itself in the body. If you believe in Mind over Matter and the Power of Suggestion, contact the Health Training and Research Center, P.O. Box 7237, Little Rock, AR 72217, and ask for information on their **Visualization Therapy** audio tapes.

39. Snake Oil

This is nothing but a good old-fashioned Echinacea Tincture and doesn't contain any snake ingredients. Traveling merchants in the Old West proved the virtues of snake oil by letting poisonous snakes and then have the tincture render the toxin harmless. The formula was given to the early settlers by native Indians and was a coveted remedy for many decades. Since the formula is an effective immune booster, it was used for virtually any disease, including cancer (which was rare at the time). It was only when greedy merchants started peddling inferior formulas that snake oil attained its tarnished reputation. Famous herbalist, Dr. Richard Schulze has designed a modern "snake oil" formula that also contains garlic oil and cayenne pepper for added potency. Echinacea Plus is available from the American Botanical Pharmacy at: 800-437-2362.

40. Vitamin K and Liver Cancer

You never see **Vitamin K** listed on nutritional labels, but don't mistake this absence for insignificance. Healthy levels of this vitamin can contribute to the prevention of osteoporosis, cavities, hardening of the arteries and cancer. Vitamin E compounds can actually kill the tumor cells involved in primary liver cancer, a common malignancy that is notoriously resistant to conventional chemotherapy. K-compounds can also kill breast and skin cancers in tissue cultures. They also enhance the cancer-fighting ability of a Vitamin A derivative, and work synergistically with Vitamin C against prostate cancer. A therapeutic dose should consist of about 500mg daily. Do not use if on prescription blood thinners, as Vitamin K also promotes normal blood coagulation. Available in most health food stores. Some foods that are high in Vitamin K include raw kale, raw Swiss chard, raw spinach and green tea.

41. Prostate Cancer

A combination of 8 herbs (PC SPES and HP8) has proven to be a promising new therapy for prostate cancer. Tests showed improvement in about 70% of patients. The formula stops the growth of the cancer and restores the body's natural ability to protect against further growth of cancer cells. Treatment under a doctor's care is recommended. For further information and product sources, do a web search for "PC SPES".

42. Stabilized Activated Oxygen

Anaerobic cancer cells cannot survive in an oxygen-rich environment. Two-time Nobel Prize winner for cancer research, Dr. Otto Warburg said: "Cancer has only one prime cause. It is the replacement of normal oxygen respiration in the body's cells by cell respiration (i.e. oxygen deficient)." Researchers now know positively that there is a direct link between decreased oxygen levels and an increase in human disease. Due to decreased air quality, shallow breathing and poor diet, the oxygen levels in the cells of most people is too low. For product information on **Stabilized Activated Oxygen Supplements** contact:

- Aquage at: 800-699-4336
- Suggested reading: *"The One-Minute Cure,"* which shows how diluted 35% food grade hydrogen peroxide can cure virtually any disease, including cancer. For more information, do a web search on this title.

43. Cantron

This all-synthetic product lowers the voltage of the cell structure by approximately 20%. The anaerobic cancer or AIDS cells convert to waste material and are eliminated. **Cantron** is non-toxic and has no known side effects. For further product information, contact:

- Medical Research Products at: 800-443-3030
- Nu-gen Nutrition at: 888-446-8184

44. Aveloz Extract

Old Amazon folk remedy. The Aveloz plant emits a type of heat that destroys vegetation around it. This property is believed to kill abnormal cell growth. Western health professionals have tested the extract and they claim it works within a short period of time. For product information, contact:

Raintree Nutrition at: www.rain-tree.com
Medical Research Products at: 800-443-
3030 Life Extension at: 800-233-2330

45. Co-enzyme Q10

Research has shown that cancer patients are deficient in **CoQ10**. The most lethal of cancers, pancreatic cancer, is linked to the greatest CoQ10 deficiency. It has been established that 100mg of CoQ10 every day is the dose required for general maintenance. The dose for cancer has not yet been established, but should most likely be higher, probably around 100-300mg a day. It has also not yet been established whether cancer is caused by a CoQ10 deficiency or whether the CoQ10 deficiency is caused by cancer. Either way, the prudent thing to do would be to supplement the diet with this beneficial antioxidant, which is also of special value to the heart and the gums. Make sure to use the potent form of CoQ10 known as Ubiquinol.

46. Borage Oil

Gammalinolic Acid (GLA) has strong therapeutic properties. Among other disorders, it helps people with PMS, heart conditions, both types of diabetes and cancer. By giving strong support to the immune system, GLA has become a promising addition to the treatment of cancer. High levels of GLA are found in cold pressed borage oil, which is available in most health food stores.

47. The Royal Rife Instrument

During the 1930s, Dr. Royal Rife developed an electronic instrument for the treatment of cancer and many other diseases. After decades of suppression an even more versatile version is now available. To protect vested interest the FDA prohibits doctors to use this effective tool. However, individuals can purchase it for personal use. Testimonials from satisfied users are very encouraging. The cost is about $2,000 (this includes a comprehensive manual). The instrument is smaller than a laptop. For more information, do a quick web search.

- Suggested reading: *"The Cancer Cure That Worked,"* by Barry Lynes

48. IP6

Scientists have discovered that cancer cells in a wide variety of cancers can be reverted back to normal cells in the presence of **IP6**. The compound is derived from cereals such as corn, sesame, wheat and rice. As a therapy, patients should take up to 8gm daily. The guidance of an

Alternative Health practitioner is suggested. The product has no side effects and is available in many health food stores or from:

- Young Again Nutrients at: 877-205-0040
- I-Herb at: 888-792-0028
- Seacoast at: 800-555-6792

49. Enzyme Therapy

Without <u>enzymes</u>, life wouldn't be possible. One of its more dramatic and largely overlooked applications is the treatment of cancer. The enzymes erode the outer shield of tumor cells, interfere with their growth and metastasis, and help the body to generate a greater amount of cancer fighting substances called "Tumor Necrosis Factor". All fresh and uncooked fruits and vegetables contain ample amounts of enzymes. For information on some of the most advanced Enzyme Supplements contact R. Garden at: 800-800-1927.

50. Pacific Yew

Extracts made from the needles of the **Pacific Yew** tree are among the most promising anti-cancer agents. Yew products can be taken internally as well as applied externally. They have been used for a wide variety of cancers, including cancer of the ovaries, lung, kidneys, colon, pancreas and leukemia. For product details contact:

Standard Process at: 800-848-5061
Become Healthy Now at: 727-461-7354

51. Breast Cancer and Anti-Perspirants

Anti-perspirants have been linked to breast cancer. When the body is prevented from purging toxins through the sweat gland at the arm pits, it deposits them in the lymph nodes. This can lead to cell mutation. Nearly all breast cancer occurs in the upper outside quadrant of the breast area. This is where lymph nodes are located.

52. Prevent Skin Cancer

One of the most feared cancers is skin cancer, as it can spread quickly to other parts of the body. Adding some **lemon peel** to the diet on a regular basis will help the skin ward off skin cancer. Also, after excessive sun bathing, rub some **cold-pressed extra virgin oil** on to the affected areas. It can help prevent tumor formation and UV damage.

53. Ellagic Acid

Clinical tests conducted at the Hollings Cancer Institute at the Medical University of South Carolina (MUSC) have shown that **Ellagic Acid**, a naturally occurring plant phenol with the highest concentrations in red raspberries, may be an extremely potent way to prevent cancer, inhibit the growth of cancer cells and arrest the growth of cancer in persons with a genetic predisposition for the disease.

54. Beets

Some people claim that after adding raw organic **beet juice** to their diet, their cancer tumors disappeared.

55. Cancer and Meat

Tests have shown that almost all cancer patients are also suffering from Acidosis and Candida (or a related fungus), although not everybody hosting that condition or organisms comes down with cancer. Meat in the diet lowers the pH level and provides an ideal breeding ground for fungus. If you have cancer or want to avoid it, stay away from (excessive) meat.

56. Immutol

Incredible natural immune booster from Norway. One hundred times more powerful than Echinacea.

- For details, contact Immunocorp at: 800-446-3063

57. Black Salve

Black salve is a relentless substance that hunts down and penetrates all abnormal skin tissue. It has been reported that it removes tumors, moles and melanoma. For product information contact: Rising Sun Health at: 406-222-9949

Vermont County Store at: 800-547-7849
Larson Century Ranch at: 509-758-5445

58. Adrenal Cancer

This is one of the deadliest cancers. Stimulates the adrenal glands to produce excess adrenaline, sky-rocketing the blood pressure. Victims usually die from a heart attack or stroke. Long term studies done by the U.S. Dept. of Health and Human Services showed that smoking 10 grams of **marijuana** kept patients in fairly good condition.

59. How to Fight Cancer and Win & How to Fight Prostate Cancer and Win

Both of these titles are important books for treatment and prevention of cancer by William L. Fischer. Available in most book stores or from Agora Health Books at: 888-821-3609.

60. Curcumin

Laboratory tests have shown that <u>curcumin</u> stops cancer cells from multiplying and destroys abnormal cells that can become cancerous. It also blocks estrogen-mimicking chemicals that promote cancer growth, and it is an antidote to Alzheimer's. Curcumin is an ingredient of the common ayurvedic spice, turmeric. Curcumin has anti-cancer properties so potent that the drug companies are in a hurry to make drug versions. It inhibits the spread of cancer cells and induces cancer cell apoptosis. Super curcumin with bioperine is available in most health food stores or from:

- Organic India at: 888-550-8332

61. Lactoferin

Researchers have found that **lactoferin** is effective against solid tumors, and it appears to work even against mestastasis, the deadliest phase of cancer and often the hardest to treat. In one study, lactoferin proved to be highly effective against pancreatic cancer. People that had been given up for dead have experienced amazing turnarounds. Doctor recommended dose is 250-500mg per day. For more information and product sources, do a quick web search for "lactoferin cancer".

62. Hp-8

Hp-8 is a rather new and unique herbal developed by Professor Waterman in Australia. Limited studies have shown it to be effective in 80-90% of prostate cases without any side effects. The majority of those taking the supplement also reported enhanced well-being, more energy, improved ability to pass urine, and considerable pain alleviation. However, due to the fact that the product is not a toxic drug, suppressive FDA rules require that no claims can be made and the product is officially sold as a supplement for general prostate health only. Based on limited research, the most effective dose is 3 tablets twice a day (total: 6 a day) on an empty stomach, between meals and any other supplements or medication. Hp-8 is available from:
- The Harmony Company at: 800-422-5518
- Pure Prescriptions at: 800-860-9538

63. Propolis

In Egypt, where **propolis** has a long history of use, studies have shown that it has strong anti-tumor activity. When test animals were given 160mg per kilogram (2.2 lbs) of body weight, propolis stopped cancer tumor formation. In animals that had already been induced with tumors, propolis was able to dramatically shrink those tumors. A similar study performed in Croatia found virtually identical results. Propolis is available in most health food stores or from:
- Durham's Bee Farm at: 901-369-9999
- The Natural Shopper at: 877-750-0300

- Stakich, Inc. at: 248-642-7023

64. Alternative Cancer Clinics

For a worldwide list of alternative cancer clinics (including U.S. and Mexico), go to:

- www.cancure.org

65. Iscador

This natural substance is derived from the mistletoe. It is injected and widely used in Europe as a complementary medicine, often in addition to conventional cancer therapies. Susan Somers claimed that she cured her breast cancer with iscador in conjunction with some radiation therapy. Available with doctor's prescription. For more information, do quick web search for "iscador".

66. Vitamin D-3

Most people are **vitamin D-3** deficient. Vitamin D-3 is extremely important for cancer prevention and recovery. Sufficient amounts, up to 10,000 IU daily (some physicians use 50,000 IU twice weekly) which causes the cancer cells to commit suicide (apoptosis). Sun exposure will not generate sufficient vitamin D-3 for a medicinal effect. Good brands are available in most health food stores.

67. Bulgaricus

This rare lactobacillus called **bulgaricus** was discovered in Russia. It is an outstanding immune stimulator that has effective cancer-fighting capabilities. Available from:

- Allergy Research Group at: 800-545-9960
- Web Vitamins at: 800-919-9122

68. Glyconutrients

The modern American diet supplies only 2 of 8 essential carbohydrates or sugars that are necessary for optimal immunity and health. Consequently, our cells mis-communicate, resulting in a myriad of disorders and diseases, including cancer. Supplementing our diet with **glyconutrients** enables our body to recover from disease and maintain health and vitality. Glyconutrients are already being successfully used for various types of cancer. Glyconutrients are not available in health food stores. For more information, do quick web search for "glyconutrients - cancer". Available from:

- Netriceuticals at: 888-852-4993
- Micro Health Solutions at: 417-863-8157

69. High pH Therapy

The **pH** in the cancer cells is increased to 8 or above. At this alkalinity the cancer cells can't survive long. For more information, so a quick web search for, "high pH therapy".

70. DIM

A natural supplement derived from broccoli and cauliflower has been found to effectively prevent and fight breast and prostate cancers. **BioResponse DIM**, which contains concentrates from these 2 plants is available in many health food stores. For more information, do a quick web search for "bioresponse DIM".

71. Fasting for Health

Fasting is a thing which most of us have forgotten. Our bodies are filled with mucous, with residuals of drugs and various kinds of toxins. Our bodies are like a machine filled with hundreds of millions of tubes. These tubes I'm talking about are our veins and cells, arteries and capillaries, etc. In most cases, they are clogged with waste products; with an oversupply of mucous material, residuals, especially alkaloids from medicinal drugs.

In order to clean the system, first of all, fast for 3 days (spring water only). If you find it too difficult, start with one day a week then work your way up to 3 days. Make sure you follow these directions:

Just before the first day of fasting, there should be a colon irrigation with a warm water enema, from 1-2 quarts. Add to this solution 1 tablespoon of raw honey and the juice of 1 lemon. On the first day of fasting, drink only spring water (no tap water) laced with honey and some lemon juice. No food should be consumed. On the second and third days, you may include some organic grapes.

The fasting is essential as it removes, or at least begins to remove, harmful toxins from your body. After 3 days of fasting, follow the simple diet below:
- For breakfast: One kind of ripe fruit, as much as you desire
- For lunch: Salads (preferably organic) with natural dressing (no hydrogenated oil, etc.)
- For dinner or supper (max 3 meals a day): Uncooked vegetables (preferably organic), no meat of any kind

The diet above should be followed for 2 days. Thereafter, a regular diet can be resumed. However, try to avoid red meat (beef, pork, etc.). A diet consisting of fish, fowl, raw fruits and vegetables, raw nuts, avocados, etc. is good. Avoid starchy cereals and breads. As a general rule, stay away from processed and too many cooked foods. They are much of the reason for our degenerative diseases and over-weight problems. Mono fruits, where one type of fruit is eaten at one meal, and raw leafy vegetables with simple natural dressing—these types of foods remove accumulated waste products that have built up in our bodies for 10-20 years, or even longer. These waste products and toxins are the basic cause for our degenerative diseases like cancer, arthritis, high blood pressure and so forth. This kind of health diet, which every person should incorporate into their lifestyle, prevents that sickness, that tragedy, that pain towards which many of us now move.

If the 3-day fast is followed once a month for a period of one year, you should notice a significant difference in your health, in the way you feel and will allow you to really understand the value of fasting. It is also suggested that those of us who now feel no specific illness or pain should also fast, so that their lives may be fuller and forestall any diseases that may be in the making. Fresh air, moderate sunshine, pure water, rest, some pleasant exercise and a relaxed state of mind should also be of concern to those in search for radiant health.

72. IV Vitamin C

Intravenous Vitamin C (IV C) has become an effective and relatively widely used cancer treatment. For more information regarding the procedure, call:
- Dr. Riordan's Clinic at: 316-682-3100
- The Whitaker Wellness Institute at: 800-488-1500
- For more information visit: drandrewlipton.com

73. Prostate Cancer

Researchers have discovered a new effective weapon for the prevention and treatment of prostate cancer called Isosilybin B, which is a component of the milk thistle. The compound is effective against both hormone dependent and hormone independent prostate cancers. For product information contact:
- Web Outpatients at: 877-438-3042
- Skye Herbals: 303-859-7585

For unrelated additional information on how to treat prostate cancer, contact:
- Health Alert
  100 Wilson Rd. #110
  Monterey, CA 93940
- (Make sure you send a self-addressed and stamped envelope, with two stamps attached to it. Just enclose a note that says "prostate".)

74. Goji Berries

In Mongolia, China, Japan and Switzerland, the Asian goji berry is now being studied for its ability to fight cancer. It has been found that the fruit, as well as extracts from its leaves, can kill many kinds of cancer in vitro. The berries contain organic germanium. This trace mineral has significant anti-cancer activity. Japanese studies indicate that organic germanium is effective in treating liver, lung, uterine, cervical and testicular cancer when combined with other treatments. It has been found to induce the production in humans of g-interferon. Interferon possesses the power to take over the hydrogen ion from cancer cells. Losing hydrogen ions can cause depression and even death of cancer cells. Besides germanium, the goji berry has other components that act against cancer. They appear to be able to depress or block the synthesis of the cancer cell's DNA, which interferes with the cell's ability to divide and this lowers the reproductive capability of the cancer cell. Soak the dried berries for half an hour and enjoy delicious goji berry juice from your blender once or twice a day. Goji berries are available from:

- Super Foods at: 800-481-5074
- Extreme Health at: 800-800-1285
- Dragon Herbs 1-888-55-TONIC

75. Epican Forte

Dr. Matthias Rath, one of the most renowned metastasis inhibition specialists, has designed a potent anti-cancer supplement called **Epican Forte**. For more information, do a quick web search for the product. Available from:

- Dr. Rath's Health Alliance at: 800-624-2442

76. The Concord Grape Cure

A strict protocol of this cure has helped many, including individuals with bone and prostate cancer. Start sipping a large bottle (24 oz.) of unsweetened, organic **Concord Grape Juice**. This product is available in most health food stores. Finish the bottle in the morning, 1-2 hours before your first meal. Avoid pork. After 4-6 weeks you should see satisfactory results. Doctors say prostate and bone cancers require more time to see results.

77. Real Butter

Real butter is a potent weapon against cancer. By "real", I mean organic, unpasteurized and from free-range animals. Avoid margarine—it's toxic! Real butter is not readily available in stores. Raw, organic butter is available from:

- Organic Pasture at: 877-729-6455
- For more information, visit: www.realbutter.com

78. Resveratrol

This is a bioflavonoid that is derived from the skin of dark grapes. It can inhibit all 3 stages of cancer. Resveratrol can also return pre-cancerous cells back to normal. For more information, do a quick web search for "resveratrol". Available from:

- Advanced Bio Nutritionals at: 800-728-2288

79. Prostate Cancer

In a recent study researchers had 25 prostate cancer patients take a daily supplement of 1.3 grams of the green tea extract **Polyphenols** (the equivalent of 12 cups of green tea). After 5 weeks, tests revealed significant drops of about 30% in PSA, HGF and VEGE. Consequently, this green tea extract is now considered to be a viable alternative for the treatment and prevention of prostate cancer.

80. Healing Cancer Naturally

One of the best and most inexpensive publications on alternative cancer therapies is the "Special Edition 2000 of the Well Being Journal: Healing Cancer Naturally" that is available from:

- The Well-Being Journal at: 775-887-1702

81. The Daniel Chapter One Program

This formula consists of 7 herbs: burdock root, sheep sorrel, Siberian ginseng, cat's claw, slippery elm, winter green and Turkey rhubarb root. It has been shown to be a potent cancer fighter, including against ovarian cancer and leukemia. For more details:

- Visit: www.danielchapterone.com
- Call: 800-504-5511

82. Activated Oxygen

The ultimate formula to saturate every cell of your body with **vital oxygen**. The originator of this formula cured herself of cancer and other diseases.

- For more information visit: www.vitalactivatedoxygen.com
- Call Vital Activated Oxygen at: 888-795-3947

83. Arginine

This amino acid is known for its wound-healing, immune-boosting and cancer-fighting abilities. It's being used on an empty stomach 2-3 times a day. **Arginine or L-arginine** is available in most health food stores.

84. MSR-3

An extraordinary immune booster. Like MGN-3, it contains the unique Arabinoxylane ingredient. Available from:

- Swanson Health Products at: 800-824-4491

85. Asparagus

Asparagus has helped many people suffering from Hodgkin's diseases, prostate, breast, lung, bladder and skin cancers, as well as leukemia and cancer of the mouth and other cancers. Results are usually achieved within 2 weeks to 6 months. The best way to take asparagus (preferably organic) is by making a puree from the cooked vegetable in a blender, and the taking 4 full tablespoons twice daily (mornings and evenings). More can't hurt and is certainly recommended for acute cases. Best taken on an empty stomach.

86. Deep Defense

A very potent combination of 2 Chinese herbs (**Astragalus and Ligustrum**) restores white blood cell count in the bone marrow and rejuvenates red blood cells. Often taken before another round of ("dead-end") chemotherapy or radiation. For more information, do a quick web search for Astragalus Ligustrum". Available as "Deep Defense" from:

- Club Natural: 800-570-8840

87. Sea Biotics

A unique marine oil that has been used for a wide-range of degenerative diseases, including lung and liver cancers. Comes in bulk bottles rather than in soft gels. For more information:
Visit: www.seabiotics.com/legend
Call: 800-572-7321 (user name: legend)

88. Cancer: Its Causes and Treatment Without Operation

According to Dr. Robert Bell, cancer is a metabolic disorder. It is caused by hypoxia, the condition whereby cells suffocate due to a lack of available oxygen. Rather than dying, cells shift their fuel source primarily away from oxygen to an anaerobic mode resembling lower plant forms of life, which thrive on a diet consisting mainly of sugars. This book reveals some of the most suppressed cancer information. Available from:

- Crusador (for $30, incl. shipping) at: 800-593-6273

89. Female Cancers

Vegetables from the "mustard family" contain a special molecule called "**I3C**". These vegetables have been used successfully in medical trials to fight female cancers like ovarian, breast, uterine and cervical cancers. **IC3** converts "bad" cancer-feeding estrogen into "good" estrogen. These mustard family vegetables include: mustard, broccoli, cauliflower, bok choy, cabbage and brussel sprouts. Eat them preferably uncooked or just slightly blanched, and organic if possible.

90. Prostate Cancer

"I was diagnosed with advanced prostate cancer, which could not be treated with surgery or radiation. My PSA level was 900.7 ng/ml. Metastatic focuses were found in a large area of my lymph gland and lumbar bone. Patients who have prostate cancer with distant metastasis in lymph glands or bones usually undergo hormone therapy with a response rate of 60-70%. However, approximately 40% of those will suffer a relapse of the condition within one year. Then no other effective therapy is considered available. I decided to use Gerson therapy at the start of the anti-hormone therapy in order to support it. In my case, it took less than a year for the anti-androgen hormone therapy to become ineffective. However, at about the same time, the Gerson therapy became effective, which resulted in a complete cure of my prostate cancer." ~ Cancer survivor, Willie L.

91. BEC5 and Non-Melanoma Skin Cancer

The product that has worked for people suffering from non-melanoma skin cancer is **BEC5**. For more information, do a quick web search for, "BEC5" sources; there are plenty of them.

92. Essential Fatty Acid Omega 3 & 6

Omega 3 and Omega 6 play a very essential role in transferring vital oxygen from the blood stream to the cells. If not transferred to the cells, oxygen-rich blood will be of little benefit. Sufficient oxygen in the cells prevents cancer as cancer cells cannot survive in an oxygen-rich environment. The fatty breast tissue requires a high concentration of Omega 6. However, due to excessive consumption of processed foods, women get very little of natural, unadulterated Omega-6. What they get is an overload of processed or deranged Omega-6. This type of Omega-6 has not only lost its ability to transfer oxygen, but it is an outright toxin that has been linked to arteriosclerosis, thickening of the blood, heart disease and cancer, especially breast cancer. The results of a major study by Dr. W. C. Willett at Harvard University showed that women with the lowest intake of unprocessed Omega-6 had the highest rate of breast cancer. Omega 3 & 6 can alleviate existing cancers, but it's more effective in the prevention of cancer. Another study by the University of Washington showed that the blood of over 200 patients who had died from heart disease contained high levels of trans linoleic acid, the deranged Omega-6 found in hydrogenated vegetable oils and processed foods.

The healthiest ratio of Omega-6 to Omega-3 is about 2 to 1 and not the reverse as is often erroneously believed. Oils with a 2 to 1 Omega-6 to Omega-3 ration are wheat germ oil, hemp oil, borage oil and evening primrose oil. The oils must be uncooked or slightly heated (warm) at the most to be of any health benefit. Processed foods and engineered oils are for suckers only. Sadly, there is one born every second. For more information:

- Visit: www.brianpeskin.com (click on "book reviews")

93. Phytonutrients

Dr. Bruce West maintains that cancer is not a localized disease, but a systemic disease that affects the entire body. That's why the entire body needs to be treated with an anticancer **phytonutrient program**, even if the patient undergoes radiation, chemo or surgery. For details, do a quick web search for, "phytonutrients & cancer". For a free copy of the encyclopedia of phytonutrients:

- Call: 800-944-6465
- For more information, call: 877-429-4858

94. Klinik St. Georg

"Six months after visiting your clinic; here is the result from the PET/CT scan! NO Malignancies! I personally thank you for your treatment, advice and cure of my prostate cancer. Please thank all the fine professionals who have helped us at your clinic. BL, USA. The website in Germany is: www.klinik-st-georg.de"

95. Low-dose Naltrexone

Naltrexone is a drug that is used to help dope addicts to withdraw from their vice. However, it has been found that a low-dose of naltrexone is also effective in treating cancer. Physicians found that approximately 60% of patients for whom conventional treatment had failed experienced considerable improvement. For more information, do a quick web search for "low-dose naltrexone – cancer".

96. Cervical Cancer

Indole-3-Carbinol (I3C) is a cruciferous vegetable that has been found to be effective against cervical cancer. In one study, in which patients were given 200-400mg of I3C daily, half the women were in complete remission after 12 weeks. I3C is also being used in the treatment of other cancers.

97. Breast Cancer and Iodine

In the 60s and 70s, iodine researcher Benjamin Eskin, M.D., pointed out the important role iodine plays in women's breast health. He found that iodine kills cancerous cells without affecting normal cells. Researchers in other countries have since confirmed Dr. Eskin's findings.

A solution of 50% Lugol's iodine and 50% of a 70% DMSO solution (for sufficient penetration), rubbed directly on the affected part of the breast and the lymph glands at the arm pits (where the cancer spreads first) has been shown to be effective. This procedure should be undertaken under the supervision of a doctor. However, don't expect much cooperation from a conventional M.D. An under-active thyroid is usually a sign of iodine deficiency. Iodine supplements are available. To find a local naturopath, contact:

- The American College for Advancement in Medicine at: 800-532-3688 (www.acam.org)
- The American Association of Naturopathic Physicians at: 866-538-2267 (www.naturopathic.org)

98. Manner Clinic

Dr. Harold W. Manner has been operating a successful clinic in Tijuana, Mexico for over 10 years, treating many different cancers. His main tool is laetrile. For more information:
- Call: 800-433-4962 or 800-248-8431
- Or visit: www.cancure.org/manner_clinic.htm

99. Pomegranates

Phenolic ellagic acid in **pomegranates** is an effective anti-cancer agent. In a study of older men with prostate cancer, the acid caused prostate cancer cells to die. One of the best pomegranate supplements is Estragranate, which is available in many health food stores or from:
- Doctor's Trust at: 800-240-6046
- iHerb at: 866-328-1171

100. Aminocare

"On Nov. 03, I was diagnosed with prostate cancer with a P.S.A of 183. An operation to the prostate could not be done because it was too large. I started taking Aminocare in mid-November along with my therapy. By March, my P.S.A. had dropped to 6, and in another month, it was below 4. I am out of the danger zone and I will continue to take Aminocare." ~ Cancer survivor, Ray N. from Cleveland, OH

- Aminocare is available from Aminocare products at: 800-856-8006 or www.aminocare.com

101. Zeolite

Zeolite, a remarkable volcanic mineral complex, has shown to be a highly effective cancer fighter. Due to its negative charge, Zeolite removes heavy metals and toxins from the body and improves alkalinity (pH level). In a study with 65 (mostly) stage 4 cancer patients, liquid Zeolite achieved a 78% cure rate and a 89% survival rate. In another study with 5 male patients of ages 51 to 69, suffering from liver cancer, prostate cancer, lung cancer, intestinal cancer and Crohn's disease, all patients experienced considerable overall improvement, increased body weight and disappearance of symptoms. Zeolite activates the p21 gene which forces the cancer cell to die.

According to Italian onocologist and author, Tulio Simoncini, M.D., *"Cancer is a Fungus"* (also title of his book), "The root of all cancer is an overgrowth of *Candida Albicans* (yeast/fungus). The accumulation of mercury and aluminum, and chemotherapy, lay the perfect foundation for the overgrowth of candida. Zeolite rids the body of heavy metals and other toxins, including candida." Noted naturopath Dr. Ede Koenig, D.Sc., Ph.D., proclaimed, "Not everybody who has candida overgrowth gets cancer, but everybody who has cancer has a candida overgrowth."

The most effective form of zeolite is powder. While liquid is considerably more expensive, it has been shown to not bind heavy metals as completely as powder. Most cancer patients take 4-6 zeolite capsules (size 00) or the equivalent in bulk powder, suspended in a liquid 3 times a day, while drinking plenty of water for adequate hydration. Zeolite is also an extraordinary overall detoxifier and health enhancer. For more information, do a quick web search for "zeolite supplements cancer". Supplemental zeolite powder is available from:
- Cutting Edge Catalog at: 800-497-9516
- Get Healthy Again at: 800-832-9755

102. Modifilan

This substance is an extract from the seaweed laminaria. Research has demonstrated **Modifilan's** remarkable ability to induce rapid cancer cell apoptosis (cancer cell death) in leukemia, stomach and colon cancer and other cancers, and to neutralize radioactive contamination of the body. Modifilan in seaweed is thought to contribute considerably to the low breast cancer rate in Japan. For more information, do a quick web search for "Limu Moui – Cancer". Available from:
- Naturo Doc at: 877-867-4743
- Modifilan Seaweed Extract at: 866-434-4039 (www.midifilan-seaweed-extract.com)
- www.naturodoc.com

103. Gingerols

Korean researchers found that gingerol, a compound in ginger, inhibits cell growth and induces cell death in human pancreatic cancer cells. Pancreatic cancer has been linked to refined sugar. For more information and product sources, do a quick web search for "gingerols".

104. DR-70 Blood Test

This is the only known test that accurately screens for 13 types of cancer at the same time. If your doctor is not familiar with this test, he/she can call AMDL, Inc. at: 714-505-4460 or email them at: mkt@amdl.com for more information.

105. Sodium Bicarbonate

Renowned Italian oncologist, Dr. Tullio Simoncini says he discovered that the cause of cancer is a common fungus, candida albicans, and that virtually any cancer can be treated with the powerful anti-fungal agent **sodium bicarbonate**. Dr. Simoncini claims that he has successfully treated many types of cancer without his patients suffering any negative side effects. For more information, visit:

- www.cancerfungus.com
- www.curenaturalicancro.com/cancer-therapy-simoncini-protocol.html
- www.curenaturalicancro.com

106. Artemesia

A humble plant that grows in Southeast Asia is a proven remedy for malaria and cancer. Chinese researchers found that the key to **artemesia**'s ability to induce cancer cell death is a peroxide linkage (two oxygen atoms hooked together) within the herb's active molecule. For more information and product sources, do a quick web search for, "Artemesia – Cancer".

107. Crinum

This herb from Vietnam has a long history as a prostate and ovarian cancer fighter. Improvement is often noticed in as little as 2 months. For more details, do a quick web search for, "Crinum – Cancer".

108. Envita Natural Medical Center of America

This treatment center – located in Scottsdale, AZ – uses over 100 natural therapies, which are applied according to the patients' needs. For more information:

- Call: 866-830-4576
- Visit: www.behealthyamerica.com

109. Wheat Grass

In his book, "How I Conquered Cancer Naturally," Eydie Mae writes that abscisic acid found in **wheat grass** is remarkably effective against all types of cancer. Freshly juiced wheat grass is available in most health food stores.

110. Natura

This Chinese encapsulated herbal formula is being used world-wide as an effective cancer remedy. For a free info-pack, call:

- American Nutriceuticals at: 941-351-9334

111. Indole-3-Carbiol (I3C)

I3C is a cruciferous vegetable extract that has been used in the prevention and treatment of various cancers. One study involved women with cervical dysplasia who were given from 200-400mg of I3C daily. After 3 months, about 50% of the women had complete regression. I3C is available in many health food stores or by mail through various Internet health shops. Cervical cancer has been linked to low levels of folate.

112. Colostrum

Colostrum is the first life-protecting secretion that a mammal produces for its newborn. Among its many benefits are extraordinary immune-boosting properties. Bovine colostrum is biologically transferrable to all mammals, including man. Since is it about 40 times more powerful than human colostrum, it is an essential part of successful alternative cancer therapy. For more information and product sources, do a quick web search for, **"Colostrum – Cancer".**

113. Selenium

This trace element has shown remarkable anti-cancer capabilities, in both prevention and treatment, including liver, prostate and breast cancer. The most effective form of **selenium** is the 100% whole food selenium, which has 100 times the bioavailability of the more commonly used sodium selenite or selenomethionine. Whole food selenium is available from:
Crusador at: 800-593-6273

114. Insulin Potentiation Therapy (IPT)

IPT was originally used to treat cancer by Dr. Perez Garcia in 1945, and has been used successfully ever since. The treatment makes the use of chemotherapy so effective that only a fraction of the normal dose is necessary, which has no or minimal side effects. The remission rate for stage 1 & 2 patients with various cancers has been about 80%. The results for the "incurable" stages 3 & 4 have been mixed. Chemotherapy doctors hate IPT because it is relatively inexpensive compared to conventional chemotherapy, and has a dramatically higher success rate. For more details and to locate treatment centers, do a quick web search for, "insulin potentiation therapy".

115. Bloodroot

This North American herb has been used by the natives for centuries to treat cancer. It contains anti-cancer/tumor properties alternative healers describe as almost unbelievable. **Bloodroot** is not a gentle healer. It relentlessly searches for and destroys cancer cells wherever it finds them throughout the entire body. The thorough removal of cancer cells may cause some initial discomfort. Bloodroot has been successfully used against breast, prostate, pancreatic and other cancers. For more information, do a quick web search for "black salve" which will provide related info, or:

- Visit: www.cancerx.org

116. The Breuss Cancer Cure

In his book, ***"The Breuss Cancer Cure,"*** Dr. Rudolph Breuss writes that he has cured over 40,000 cancer patients with a 42-day special vegetable juice only therapy. Purchase his book for complete details.

The Breuss juice calls for these vegetables and ratios: red beet (9), carrots (3), celery roots (3), potatoes (3) and black radish (1). All vegetables should be organic and must be juiced in their raw and unpeeled state. The regiment calls for this juice only and nothing else for 42 days. Any protein consumed during that time may doom the remedy to failure. This actually sounds more difficult than it really is and his book gives complete guidance and details.

Natural health guru, Dr. John Heinerman recommends the juices of beet, cabbage, apricot, wheat grass and barley grass as remedies against cancer. Details can be found in his book titled, "Heinerman's Encyclopedia of Healing Juices".

The healthiest and most effective juice for cancer therapy is made with a twin gear juicer rather than the conventional grinding-disc type juicer which tears and shreds. Twin gears extract the juice by pressing and crushing. This action is gentler on the enzymes, breaks down the cells walls for more thorough assimilation, extracts more minerals and produces more of a better tasting juice, with the pulp almost dry. For more information, do a quick web search for "twin gear juicers".

If you use a conventional juicer, be aware that some of the most nutritious juice is left in the pulp, which is usually thrown away. A pulp press can extract most of the juice that is then left in the pulp. For more information, do a quick web search for "juicer pulp press".

117. Optimum Health

For information regarding a 3-week wheat grass, raw food, etc. detoxification program at a very reasonable cost:

- Visit: www.optimumhealth.org

118. Amas Blood Test

This test will detect about 99% of all cancers up to 1.5 years earlier than the much more intrusive and dangerous conventional tests. For details, do a quick web search for, "Amas Blood Test". Another noted test is the DR-70 blood test (mentioned earlier in this book) that can screen for 13 types of cancers at the same time.

119. Prostate Cancer Info

For a free prostate flyer describing successful prostate cancer protocol, send a self-addressed and stamped (2 stamps) envelope to:

- Health Alert
  100 Wilson Rd.,
  Monterey, CA 93940
- Make sure you write "PROSTATE" in large letters in the left lower corner.

120. 3-BrPA

A compound called 3-BrPA, pioneered by Dr. Ko, has been found to be especially effective against liver cancer. For more details, do a quick web search for "3-BrPA" and "John Hopkins Liver Cancer Center".

121. Avemar

Avemar is an extract of fermented wheat germ. It has been proven to be effective against all types of cancer and alleviates the deadly effects of radiation and chemotherapy. It is an extraordinary immune system enhancer. For more details, do a quick web search for "Avemar".
Available from:

- Betterlife.com at: 800-317-7150
- Fubao Health Store at: 866-883-8226

122. Cranberries

Laboratory tests have shown that disease-fighting flavonoids in cranberries have the ability to fight and destroy prostate cancer cells.

123. Reishi

Reishi, also known as Ling Zhi, Ling Zhih and Ganoderma Lucidum, is one of the most coveted oriental herbs. It is used for a vast array of disorders and diseases. Alternative health professionals use it extensively for all types of cancers, including breast, prostate, lung, liver and pancreatic cancer. Unpolluted and effective reishi is available from:

- Quantum Nutrition at: 877-987-8468 (www.qnhshop.com) / v-caps
- Health Products USA at: 978-290-4465 (www.healthproductsusa.net) / powder in caps
- Mountain Rose Herbs at: 800-879-3337 (www.mountainroseherbs.com)/ sliced mushroom

To prepare Ling Zhih tea, cut the mushroom into very small pieces (as small as possible). Simmer about 8gms (a little more than ¼ oz.) in 4 cups of spring water for 30 minutes on low heat. Don't use metal pots; glass or coated/enameled containers are preferable. You should end up with about 2 cups. Drink half a cup twice daily. If too bitter, sweeten with stevia or **raw** honey. Keep your mushrooms stored in a cool, dark place. Some users may get a little sleepy after consumption; if necessary, take a small nap.

124. Acai

The **acai** berry grows in the Amazon rainforest in Brazil and is one of the most nutritious fruits on Earth. A study by the University of Florida and published in the Journal of Agriculture and Food Chemistry in January of 2006 showed that certain components in the berry trigger self-destruction (apoptosis) of cancer cells. Acai juice is not recommended, as it is pasteurized, this greatly diminishing the effectiveness of the product. Organic, raw, freeze-dried acai powder is a preferable choice and is available from:

- Healthy Choice Naturals at: 800-541-6779 (www.healthychoicenaturals.com)
- Sambazon at: 877-726-2296 (www.sambazon.com)
- For more information, do a quick web search for "Acai Cancer" and Acai Extract"
- Also note that grapes, mangos and guavas are known cancer killers

125. Bio Response DIM

Bio Response DIM is a vegetable extract. A Wayne State University study found that the compound stimulates self-destruction (apoptosis) of prostate cancer cells and inhibits the growth of new blood vessels in prostate cancer tissue. Although the study focused on prostate cancer, causes and treatment for breast cancer are quite similar. BioResponse DIM is available from:

- BioResponse Nutrients at: 877-312-5777 (www.bioresponse.com)
- For more information, do a quick web search for "BioResponse DIM"

126. Breast Cancer

Research by immunologist, Dr. Kris McGarth of Northwestern University in Illinois has linked the use of underarm antiperspirants that contain aluminum to breast cancer. When toxins that are normally expelled through underarm sweat glands are trapped, they tend to migrate to adjacent breast tissue where they can cause cancer. A preferable alternative to an antiperspirant would be a deodorant.

127. Urine and AMAS Cancer Tests

Early warning is critical in successfully treating cancer. **Urine and AMAS (blood) cancer tests** are amazingly accurate, non-intrusive, simple and inexpensive. For more details, do a quick web search for "Urine Cancer Test" and "AMAS Cancer Test".

128. Select Cancers

The World Research Foundation collects **research of natural remedies** for many diseases. Information on cancer of the following organs is available at a very reasonable cost: bladder, bone, breast, cervix, colon, kidney, leukemia, liver, lung, lymphoma, ovarian, pancreatic, prostate, skin, uterus and more. For more information:

- Call: 928-284-3300
- Visit: www.wrf.org

129. Pau D'Arco, Chaparral and Red Clover Tea

"In April 1983, I became very ill. After being tested and x-rayed by my own doctor and a specialist, I was told I had cancer. I was immediately sent to a San Francisco hospital, where I was extensively tested and x-rayed. I received the same diagnosis and the cancer had progressed and enveloped the lining of my right lung. Several doctors reviewed my case. A few days later, I was told there was no treatment for this type of cancer. I insisted that I be released from the hospital with appointments to return.

My first return appointment was on May 17, 1983. I wasn't any better and was taking pills for pain. My next appointment was on June 14, 1983. More tests and x-rays were made. At this time, the pills had to be increased for the severe pain I was in. My doctor told me that several doctors had evaluated my case and didn't think I had over 6 months to live. During the conversation, I asked the name of my type of cancer. He said it was the same type Steve McQueen died of (mesothelioma – usually related to asbestos exposure), and that it was very fast-acting cancer. I told the doctor that I was going to attempt to treat myself through nutrition or any other method I could find. He said, "sure, anything".

It wasn't until the first week of July 1983, while visiting a friend that I learned about the combination of Pau D'Arco bark, chaparral leaf and red clover herb tea. His wife had heard that I had only a short time to live. She told me she had something that may cure me in 30 days. I had my doubts, but I was willing to try anything. When back home, I immediately started drinking tea made with these three herbs. (Pau D'Arco is also known as taheebo, ipe roxo and purple lapacho). Within 24 hours, I had no more pain. A few days later after taking the tea and being on a very nutritious (primarily raw) diet, I began having excessive bowel movements which lasted about 2.5 days. Immediately I started to feel better. By August 2, 1983, I had been taking the tea for three weeks and two days. More tests and x-rays were taken to see how far the cancer had progressed. The doctor found that I no longer had cancer. My lung was clear. My amazed doctor asked me what I had done to cure myself. When I told him of the teas, he cautioned me not to continue taking them (which of course I ignored). On November 1, 1983, I had my last checkup and had no more cancer. I have told several people that I had terminal cancer how I was cured. They tried it and were also cancer-free in a short time. I feel that the combination of the three teas and eating simple, nutritious foods is what healed my body. I'm glad now that my doctors considered chemo and radiation ineffective for my type of cancer. Had I undergone those treatments, I'm sure they would have done me in." ~ cancer survivor, Robert A.

130. Urine Therapy

No matter how unbelievable this story may sound to you, the truth is this simple approach to cancer and hundreds of other ailments has an old history and is one of the most extraordinary and successful disease treatments the world has ever seen. Since there is no money in this therapy, it is being kept out of the spotlight by special interest. Dr. Evagelos Danopoulos of Greece found that urea found in urine has anti-cancer properties that disrupt the cancer cells' metabolic activities. **Urine therapy** is being used to treat cancers of the lungs, liver, breast, cervix, eyes, and skin among others. For more information, do a quick web search for "urine therapy cancer".

- Suggested reading: "Your Own Perfect Medicine," by Martha Christy. ISBN# 0963209116

131. Modified Citrus Pectin (MCP)

MCP contains a shorter sugar chain that interferes with the ability of the cancer cells to proliferate. Modified citrus pectin has been used successfully against cancers of the prostate, breast, colon, and lung among others. For more information, do a quick web search for, "Modified Citrus Pectin MCP Cancer". Available from:

- Bio Essence at: 510-215-5588

132. Cholesterol

An extensive 1980 French study showed that the cancer rate increases as **cholesterol** falls below 200. Cholesterol, which is produced by the liver (including LDL), is a vital body chemical needed by every organ in the body, especially the brain.

133. Cinnamon & Honey

Research in Australia and Japan has revealed that advanced cancer of the stomach and bones can be cured successfully with **cinnamon and raw honey**. Patients took 1 tablespoon of raw honey mixed with 1 teaspoon of cinnamon powder for 1 month, 3 times a day.

134. Coconut Oil

"After having had a mastectomy, lumpectomy and chemotherapy for breast cancer, I was diagnosed with a skull full of cancer just a few months later, and was given 2 months to live. At that time I came across some research about clinical trials for AIDS in the Philippines using **coconut oil**. I figured if coconut oil can boost the immune system and cure AIDS, it might work for my cancer. I started taking 3 to 4 tablespoons of organic extra virgin coconut oil a day plus whatever I used in preparing my meals. I would add it to my oatmeal in the morning, put it in my hot chocolate and cook my meals in it. I also snacked on fresh coconut and drank fresh coconut milk. When my doctors monitored the cancer six months later, to their complete surprise, the cancer had gone into remission. Today I continue to use this miracle organic extra virgin coconut oil and I'm cancer free!" ~ cancer survivor, Julie Figueroa

135. Artemisinin

This cancer remedy is a derivative of the Wormwood herb. Studies at the University of Washington showed **artemisinin** to be effective against a wide variety of cancers, especially colon cancer and leukemia. In one publicized case, a patient suffering from leimyosarcoma with mets to the liver saw his tumors disappear within 4 weeks.

136. Pao Pereira

Dr. Mirko Beljanski's laboratory tests have shown that this extract from a Brazilian tree effectively suppresses proliferation of Cancer, Leukemia and HIV cells. Available from:

- Natural Source International at: 888 308-7066,
- Tropilab at: 727 344-7608

137. Exercise with Oxygen Therapy (EWOT)

Cancer cells cannot survive in an oxygen-rich environment. **EWOT** requires a small oxygen bottle or an oxygen separator and a small stationary piece of exercise equipment like a treadmill. In contrast to conventional exercise, EWOT is capable of not only enriching the blood with oxygen, but quickly transfers the oxygen from the blood to every cell of the body. For therapeutic purposes an output of about 95% pure oxygen and a flow rate of 8 to 10 lpm (liters per minute) is necessary. The least expensive short term way would be the use of small oxygen bottles. In the long run, oxygen separators/generators would be more economical. A good machine with the above mentioned output costs around $2,000. Chemotherapy depletes the body of oxygen, that's why patients who choose to go this route should also do EWOT. Unfortunately, virtually no mainstream doctor will recommend this to cancer patients. Vaccinations, smoking, major surgery and x-rays will also deplete the body's oxygen level. EWOT is also a very beneficial exercise for healthy people. For more information, do a quick web search for:

- "EWOT Training", then click on "Gold Medal Package" (that's the most suitable package).

138. Beta-1, 3D Glucan

Beta Glucan is a powerful immune boosting product. Whether you want to prevent cancer or want to heal from it. It is very important to get your immune system in cancer-fighting shape. Available from:

- Transfer Point at: 855-877-8220

- Visit: www.ancient5.com

139. Immpower AHCC

This formula is made from specially cultivated mushrooms. Its effective ingredient is activated hexose correlate compound (AHCC). The formula has shown to effectively induce cancer remission in human clinical trials. Also noticed were energy surges and alleviation of chemo side effects. A similar product called NK-9(, is available for pets). For more information and product sources, do a quick web search for "Immpower" and "NK-9".

140. Maple Syrup and Baking Soda

An effective and inexpensive cancer treatment that was pioneered by Dr. Jim Kelmun. The formula can be made from two simple household items. Mix one part of aluminum-free **baking soda** with 3 parts of **organic maple syrup**. Heat gently (not over 120 degrees) on a low flame while stirring for 5-10 minutes until the ingredients form a homogenous mass. After cooling, take 3 teaspoons every day between meals. Cancer cells thrive on sugar, but cannot survive in an alkaline and oxygen-rich environment. The maple syrup is the bait, but the baking soda, due to its alkalinity (high pH level) and ability to introduce more oxygen into the cancer cells, will kill the cancer cells. In clinical tests terminal cancer patients have experienced a cure or improvement rate of over 90%. Work virtually for all types of cancer, including lung and breast cancer.

141. Prostate Cancer

One of the more innovative and successful **prostate cancer treatments** is surgery and radiation-free high intensity focused ultrasound (HIFU). It boasts a 94% success rate with minimal temporary side effects. For more information, do a quick web search for "HIFU Prostate Cancer".

Be very leery about prostate needle biopsies. The up to 12 needle punctures create passages for cancer cells, thus spreading the cancer to adjacent tissue. Also, needle biopsies are not reliable, possibly missing the cancerous tissue giving the patient the false impression of being cancer free.

142. Nickel and Breast / Prostate Cancer

For some not quite understood reason, breast tissue and the prostate attract the toxic metal nickel. Harmful bacteria thrive on nickel. Thus these sites become the dumping ground for bad bacteria and eventually promote cancer. Stainless steel pots and pans especially dental amalgam fillings are the main reasons for nickel poisoning. The common seaweed kelp is effective in eliminating nickel from breast tissue and the prostate gland. Kelp is available in most health food stores or online.

143. Starve Your Cancer

Eliminate processed foods, pasteurized dairy products, meat and most cooked foods (only blanch your vegetables if you can't eat them raw). Also stop eating simple carbohydrates like white flour and rice, pasta, refined white sugar and artificial sweeteners, especially corn syrup. We find corn syrup in hundreds of processed foods, ice creams and beverages. Read labels. These foods are acid-forming, deprive the cells of oxygen and feed cancer cells. Instead, eat enzyme-rich raw organic fruits and vegetables, especially green leafy chlorophyll-rich vegetables. Avocados, raw cauliflower and broccoli also have cancer-inhibiting properties. Prescription drugs, coffee, and radiation from wireless phones and computers also elevate acidity.

144. Additional Cancer Therapies and Information

Visit: www.cancertutor.com for additional insight on alternative cancer treatments.

145. Use Several Therapies Simultaneously

Different people have different body chemistries. What works for one individual doesn't necessarily work for another. You may not have time to try various remedies one after another. Therefore, it is prudent to use several promising remedies, at least 2 or 3, simultaneously.

146. The Dr. Gonzalez Regimen

This regimen is based on a strict organic and natural diet, detoxification and pancreatic enzymes. It works for virtually all cancers. When the enzymes are taken between meals in sufficient qualities, they are extra-effective and actually kill cancer cells. Even hopeless pancreatic cancer patients experienced remarkable improvements. According to Dr. Gonzales, the over success rate of his regimen is about 80%. For more information:

- Visit: www.dr-gonzalez.com

147. Cancer and Statin Drugs

If you are fighting cancer it is imperative that do not take cholesterol-lowering statin drugs. These drugs depress cellular oxygen levels which in turn promotes cancer.

148. Issels Treatment

This treatment was pioneered by German doctor Joseph M. Issels some 50 years ago. It combines various natural therapeutic approaches (including a vaccine developed from the patient's own blood), and is often used in conjunction with conventional cancer therapies. Issels treatment is said to have been successful in hopeless cases, and the cure rate is over 80%. Several Issels treatment centers are now operating in the U.S. For more information, do a quick web search for "Issels Treatment".

149. Concentrated Flax Hull Lignans

These lignans are a real wonder-food which not only cause cancer cells to commit mass suicide, but also fights AIDS, diabetes, heart disease, enlarged prostate and other disorders. Available from: (www.aidshivawareness.org)

150. Skin Cancer

"Curaderm" is an extract from the Australian eggplant. This top-rated skin cancer treatment has helped thousands of people since its debut in 1990. According to user surveys, when topically applied for 12 weeks it has a nearly 100% cure rate without harming healthy tissue. For more information and product sources do a quick web search for "Curaderm Skin Cancer".

151. Particular Types of Cancer

Dr. Ralph Moss has researched virtually all types of cancer and is now offering some 200 extensive reports (several hundred pages) on various types of cancer and how to best treat them. The reports are not cheap, costing approximately $300-$500 each, but in acute cases, they are well worth the cost. For more details:

- Visit: www.cancerdecisions.com

152. Mushrooms

A recent medical study showed that regular **edible mushrooms**—besides having an anti-microbial and antioxidant effect—also inhibit the growth of cancer cells.

153. One Answer to Cancer

Dr. William Kelley was a luminary among holistic health professionals. His do-it-yourself book, "One Answer for Cancer" is a classic. He was the physician who cured actor Steve McQueen from mesothelioma. When McQueen accounted, "I'm going to blow the lid of this cancer racket," he was silenced with a fatal blood clotting injection after surgery to remove gobs of encapsulated dead cancer cells. For details regarding Dr. Kelley's regimen, do a quick web search for: "Dr. Kelley One Answer to Cancer".

154. Miracle Mineral Supplement MMS

MMS has often been called "The Miracle Mineral" of the 21st Century. It has been used successfully against many serious diseases, including most cancers, AIDS and leukemia. For more information, do a quick we search for "MMS Cancer Treatment".

155. Essential Myrrh Oil

Researchers at Rutgers University found that **myrrh** has potent anti-cancer properties that are effective against many cancers, including breast and prostate cancer and malignant brain tumors. Traditional use calls for a few drops of myrrh oil being massaged into the foot sole and on the part of the body that is closest to the cancer. The oil should be organic and cold pressed. For more information and myrrh oil sources, do a quick web search for "essential myrrh oil cancer treatment".

156. Blue Green Algae

Researchers have discovered that **blue green algae** contain extraordinary anti-cancer activity. In a test, 51 out of 65 stage 4 cancer patients became cancer free on a blue green algae regiment. An excellent blue green algae product derived from pristine Klamath Lake in Oregon is available from:

- Quantum Nutrition at: 866-627-1577
- For more information, do a quick web search for: "blue green algae cancer"

157. Cesium Chloride

Cesium chloride is one of the most alkaline elements. Nobel Prize winner, Otto Warburg, showed that cancer thrives in anaerobic (without oxygen) or acidic environments. When calcium is absorbed by cancer cells, it raises the pH level and oxygen content of the cells and the cancer cells die. Cesium chloride combined with DMSO as a carrier makes cesium chloride even more effective. However, cesium chloride causes some potassium depletion and should be taken only with potassium supplements. Furthermore, supervision of a health care specialist is recommended. Available from these websites:

- www.thewolfeclinic.com/cesium.html
- www.rainbowminerals.net/cesiumPH.htm
- For more information, do a quick web search for, "cesium chloride cancer"

158. Skin Cancer

"I had a cancer on my face for 5 years, about the size of a pencil eraser. For a cure, I mixed 1 teaspoon of baking powder and 1 teaspoon of honey, then applied to the cancer for two weeks, changing the dressing every other day. The treatment cured the cancer. It has been 24 years and the cancer has not come back. I learned this from a Baptist missionary who cured a similar cancer on his wife's lip. The cancer was the size of a dime. The "doctors" had wanted to remove the cancer by taking a part of her lip off. Make sure the honey you use is pure, local, natural raw honey that has not been heated." ~ cancer survivor, A. Brown.

159. World Research Foundation

This non-profit health information network maintains an extensive library system that contains information dating back to the 1600s. Researchers gather traditional as well as the latest alternative and natural therapies from books, periodicals and other forms of literature on virtually any disease and health problem, including cancer. The fees to obtain all available literature on a vast spectrum of illnesses and how to treat them are more than reasonable. For details, contact:

- World Research
  Foundation 41 Bell Rock
  Plaza Sedona, AZ 86351
- Tel: 928-284-3300
- www.wrf.org

160. Tetracycline

A relatively safe drug that is usually used as an antibiotic, however, **tetracycline** has been found to be also surprisingly effective in inhibiting bone cancer and the untreatable asbestos induced lung cancer mesothelioma. This inexpensive drug will not necessarily cure cancer, but it can buy time for other therapies to take hold. As an antibiotic, tetracycline will damage the beneficial flora and therefore the diet should be supplemented with a probiotic. Guidance of a naturopath is recommended.

161. Vitamin K2

A study published in the *Journal of Cancer Research* found that **vitamin K2** is effective against leukemia, ovarian and pancreatic cancer. Recommended dose is 50-90mg a day with a meal.

162. Electromagnetic Pollution

Dirty electricity in the form of electromagnetic frequencies (EMFs) have invaded virtually every home and office, creating havoc with our immune system. This man-made radiation—emitted from computers, TVs, cell phones, fluorescent light, appliances, power lines, etc.—has been linked to birth defects, miscarriages, pre-term delivery, stillbirth and many other types of cancer, especially breast cancer. All humans, especially cancer patients, should protect themselves against this serious health hazard. To find suitable protection, do a quick web search for "EMF Radiation Protection".

- Suggested reading: *"More Silent Fields,"* by Donna Fisher, which explains the problems and gives practical advice on EMF protection.

163. Triphala

A combination of three ayurvedic herbs with remarkable healing properties, one of them with the capability of inducing cell death in tumor cells while sparing normal cells. A study by the

University of Pittsburgh Cancer Institute suggests that <u>Triphala</u> may be able to even fights dreaded pancreatic cancer. Triphala is taken as a tonic by stirring 2-3 grams of the powder into hot water and drinking it throughout the day. Since the tonic doesn't taste the greatest, Triphala is also available as tablets or in capsules. For more information and product sources, do a quick web search for "Triphala Cancer" and "Triphala Tablets".

164. Stage IV Cancer Treatment

Dr. James Forsythe has been treating stage IV cancer patients in Reno, NV, with natural supplement poly-MVA therapy since 2004, with encouraging results. For more details:

- Visit: www.drforsythe.com

165. Mistletoe

Mistletoe has become a more well-known cancer treatment since Suzanne Somers cured her breast cancer with this yuletide herb. It is widely used in Europe for stomach, colon, lung and breast cancer while revitalizing the immune system and helping to repair DNA damage caused

by cancer. However, mistletoe therapy is unsuitable for self-treatment as it is usually given by injection. The most popular mistletoe therapy brand is Iscador (which I've talked about earlier in this book). It has minimal side-effects and can be used in conjunction with other therapies. Iscador requires a subscription and the supervision of a health care professional. Your physician can order Iscador directly from the manufacturer Weleda by:

- Calling: 800-241-1030
- Visiting: usa.weleda.com/medicine/integrative_cancer_therapy/index.aspx
- For more information, do a quick web search for "Iscador Mistletoe Therapy"

166. The Burzynski Clinic

Dr. Stanislaw Burzynski has been successfully treating cancer patients in his Houston clinic for over 30 years. His antineoplaston therapy converts cancer cells back to normal cells. The FDAhas tried to shut him down for decades, but due to public support and political pressure, our "consumer agency" has been forced to grudgingly keep its hands off Dr. Burzynski. His clinic offers alternative treatment for some different types of cancer. The success rate for the most common type of child brain cancer—astrocytomas—is 93%, and the prostate cancer success rate is 91%. The success rate of other types of cancer is approximately 60-70%. Dr. Burzynski has been subject to much harassment by the FDA. For more information:

- Call the clinic's free consultation line at: 713-335-5667 or 800-714-7181
- Visit: www.burzynskiclinic.com

167. Growth Hormone Milk

If you are battling cancer, it is imperative that you refrain from drinking milk from cows that have been injected with the genetically engineered bovine growth hormone rbGH. This hormone ends up in the milk and has been linked to a variety of cancers. Bovine growth hormone milk is commonly found on supermarket shelves.

168. How to Treat Almost Any Cancer at Home for $5.12 a Day

This easy-to-read 40-page booklet by Bill Henderson gives intriguing information on how to treat cancer inexpensively at home using natural remedies. Contains supplement/diet guidelines, case histories, alternative cancer clinics in the U.S. and the opportunity to sign up for a 'cancer coach'. The coaching is done by telephone as often as necessary. Available in book stores (ISBN# 978-1-61539-952-9) or online for about $20. Highly recommended.
 www.beating-cancer-gently.com

169. Root Canals

Root canals can be a breeding ground for microbes and a major cause for a compromised immune system. They have been linked to various types of cancer, especially breast cancer. Records revealed that 98-100% of breast cancer patients had root canals. Teeth with root canals usually have to be safely removed to successfully fight the cancer. If you have cancer and a root canal, consult with a biological dentist. Regular dentists will not be able to help; they may even ridicule you. Even if the cancer is cured with alternative therapy, if the teeth aren't taken care of, the cancer may recur. To find a biological dentist in your area, do a quick web search for "biological dentists". For more information, do a quick web search for "root canals cancer". Biological dentists generally also advise cancer patients to have all amalgam (mercury) fillings replaced as they also are an immune system suppressant.

170. Vitalsail

This effective medication is derived from the Taiwanese mountain mushroom, Antrodia Camphorata. The mushroom contains an especially high amount of cancer-fighting compounds called triterpenoids. A 2008 study revealed that this mushroom not only prevented breast, lung and bladder cancer as well as leukemia, but also reversed the cancers. On the negative side, **Vitalsail** is a little on the expensive side. A one-week supply (capsules) will cost about $140, but may be well worth it. Vitalsail is available in the U.S. from Khong Corporation:

- Call: 877-889-8968
- Visit: www.myasianstore.com
- For more information, do a quick web search for "Vitalsail Cancer"

171. Bisphenol A (BPA)

This toxin is widely found in plastic food containers and in liners of metal food cans. This pervasive toxin can alter the function of over 200 genes. BPA has been linked to reproductive damage and various cancers, especially breast and prostate cancer. The FDA declared BPA "safe" although the FDA's own scientific advisory board and the National Institute of Health (NIH) disagreed. Avoid foods that come in plastic containers. Use only glass or ceramic bottles to store food. Plastics #3 and #7 are especially toxic. If you must use plastic, stick to plastics #1, #2 and #5. They are considered more inert. The numbers are found in a triangle on the bottom of plastic containers. Avoid canned food; they are 'dead' foods with minimal nutrition anyway. Try to always cook with fresh ingredients.

172. Transfer Points Beta-1 3D Glucan

One of the most effective booster of the immune system, which is crucial for successfully fighting any type of cancer. The recommended amount is one capsule per 50 lbs. of body weight in the morning on an empty stomach. For details and product sources, do a quick web search for, "Beta-1 3D Glucan Transfer Point".

173. The Overnight Cancer Cure (OCC)

This rather inexpensive, safe and innovative cancer treatment is officially still considered "experimental" although it has already been used effectively for several years, even in cases of advanced cancer. OCC does not kill cancer cells, but instead reverts the cancer cells to normal cells. For more information, do a quick web search for "Overnight Cancer Cure".

174. Raspberries and Pineapple

Researchers have found that raspberries and pineapple both contain acids with distinct anti-cancer properties. While pineapple is usually always available, raspberries are seasonal. However, cancer patients can obtain raspberry extracts from:
- Herbal Extracts Plus at: 877-220-4719 (vegi-caps)
- Honey Comb Vitamins at: 877-220-4719 (liquid concentrate)

175. Cell Forte

This combination of Inositol and IP-6 increases the body's natural killer cells (NKs) and strengthens cellular defenses. NKs destroy cancer cells without harming normal cells. Available from:
- Evitamins at: 888-222-6065
- Visit: www.evitamins.com
- For more information, do a quick web search for "cell forte"

176. Immune Assist and Transfer Factor Plus

These are two effective natural supplements that proliferate NKs in the body. Available from:
- Aloha Medicinals at: 877-835-6091
- Visit: www.alohamedicinals.com

- Immune Assist and Transfer Factor Plus are used in conjunction with Avemar (page 39) and Cell Forte.

177. Antibiotics and Breast Cancer

A study published in *The Journal of the America Medical Association* indicated that women who take antibiotics have an increased risk of breast cancer. Another similar study conducted in Finland reached the same conclusion.

178. Protocel

This remarkable formula is effective for virtually any type of cancer. It is based on Dr. Otto Warburg's discovery that cancer cells are anaerobic and cannot survive in an aerobic (oxygen-rich) environment. Protocel kills cancer cells as well as other abnormal and diseased cells by fragmenting them while not harming normal cells. Testimonials from users have been overwhelming; Protocel (2 formulas 23 and 50) has been so effective that it was outlawed as a cancer therapy. However, it recently re-emerged as a general "health tonic". Consequently, no direction on how to take the formula most effectively as a cancer treatment can be given by the manufacturer or merchants. However, in her book *"Outsmart Your Cancer,"* by Tanya Harter Pierce, the author shares with readers extensive information on Protocel with detailed user instructions. Please note that hormone-blocking drugs will decrease the effectiveness of Protocel if taken during the regimen.

For more information:

- Visit: www.outsmartyourcancer.com

An interesting website from user testimonials is:

- www.alternativecancer. com

You can purchase Protocel from:

- Renewal & Wellness at: 888-581-4442 (www.webnd.com)
- Vitamin Depot at: 330-634-0008 (www.yourvitamindepot.com)

179. Hemp Seeds and Hemp Seed Oil

Hemp seeds and hemp seed oil contain the essential fatty acids (EFAs) Omega 3 & 6 in the ideal proportion of 1 part of Omega 3 to 2.5 parts of Omega 6. Essential means that the body cannot manufacture it, it has to come from a person's diet. Most people are grossly deficient in these two heat-sensitive EFAs. They are crucial for transferring oxygen from the blood to the cells, which is an especially vital function for cancer patients. Both products are available in most health food stores.

180. Prostate Cancer Drugs

Testosterone-blocking drugs for prostate cancer (Lupron, etc.) can make the prostate cancer grow faster even though the PSA may decrease.

181. Neutralizing Chemo and Radiation Side Effects

Goji berry juice has been found to help neutralize the damage caused by chemo therapy and radiation. Commercially available goji juice is not recommended as it is usually pasteurized and processed in other nutrient-diminishing ways. Soak them for a few hours, then mix with spring water for a delicious drink in a blender. Add some Xylitol or raw honey if a sweetener is needed. Have a glass 2-4 times a day. Dried goji berries are available in most health food stores.

182. Nutritional Guidelines

Regardless of what type of cancer you are afflicted with, your first line of defense is super nutrition. Include plenty of raw (preferably organic) dark green vegetables in your diet like spinach, kale, Swiss chard, parsley, collards, broccoli, dark leaf lettuce, etc. Also of value are brussels sprouts, celery, raw almonds (beware—**virtually all "raw"** almonds are irradiated these days. Proper raw almonds are available from Organic Pastures at: (877-729-6455), apricot kernels, black walnuts, sprouted grains, chlorella, spirulina, blue green algae, berries, green tea, papaya, pineapple, beets, asparagus, mushrooms, tomatoes, cucumbers, peppers, garlic, onions, carrots, etc. Make sure you avoid refined sugar, artificial sweeteners, refined oils, margarine, white flour products, coffee, processed cheese, red meat, fat-free dairy products, pasteurized/homogenized milk, sugary soft drinks and all processed foods.

183. Avocados and Prostate Cancer

Research at the University of California revealed that the high content of carotenoids, zeaxanthin, alpha-carotene, beta-carotene, Vitamin E and monounsaturated fatty acids in **avocados** are effective against prostate cancer. Mixed with a little cold-pressed hemp seed oil, and few spices if desired, will make the therapy even more effective.

184. Nutrition 2000

This business assists people with prostate cancer through alternative non-toxic treatments. For more information:
Visit: www.nutrition2000.com

185. Aglycon Sapogenin (AGS)

AGS is a ginseng extract that has been found by a UCLA study to be effective against cancer, including multiple drug resistant cancers by inducing cancer cell apoptosis. An AGS-based formula called *Careseng Oral Solution* is available from:

- Pegasus at: 604-303-9952
- Eco Nugenics Inc. at: 800-308-5518
- For more information, do a quick web search for: "Aglycon Sapogenin sources"

186. Modified Citrus Pectin (MCP)

MCP is an extract from the pulp and rinds of citrus fruits. The extract's short sugar chain initiates a chemical reaction that has the potential to stop metastases and even kill cancer cells. The most popular MCP is called PectaSol, which is available in vegetable caps and bulk powder. For more information, do a quick web search for "PectaSol".

187. Force C

This potent formula is a natural Aglycon Sapogenin extract derived from Panax Ginseng. **Force C** inhibits cancer growth in minor doses and causes cancer cells to die in higher doses. Available from:

- Health Secrets, Inc. at: 313-561-6800 (www.healthsecretsusa.com)
- Women's International Pharmacy at: 877-896-7050 or 623-214-7100

188. Breast and Prostate Cancer

Breast Defend is an advanced formula for the prevention and treatment of breast cancer. Part of this synergistic formula are three medicinal mushrooms and DIM that stop the proliferation of cancer cells. For more information and product sources, do a quick web search for "BreastDefend". ProstaCaid is a formula similar to BreastDefend, but also contains other natural ingredients to support male hormonal balance and cellular health. For more information:

- Econugenics 800-308-5518 www.econugenics.com

189. Mouth Cancer

This type of cancer is usually brought on by smoking and it can spread to nearby lymph nodes. The conventional treatment is the surgical removal of the afflicted tissue. However, many individuals have gotten rid of the lesion with 35% food-grade hydrogen peroxide. With a Q-tip, rub the liquid into the lesion twice a day. Expect a little sting. The cancer usually disappears within 3 months.

190. Never Be Sick Again – Health is a Choice, Learn How to Choose It (by Raymond Francis)

"I am a 10-year cancer survivor. I have had surgery, radiation and chemotherapy. None of it worked. For the past 8 years I have stayed alive on alternative therapy. As a result, I have read over 100 books on health. Francis's book has put all the bits and pieces together in one volume. For the first time I have been able to understand the biochemistry of my illness and I now follow a path which has greatly diminished my illness and has brought me close to remission. The information on what to do is comprehensive. More importantly is the extensive information on what not to do and things to avoid. I recommend this book to everyone, particularly to those people with a chronic illness. I wish that I would have had this book 10 years ago." ~ an ecstatic reader and cancer survivor

II. Survivor Stories

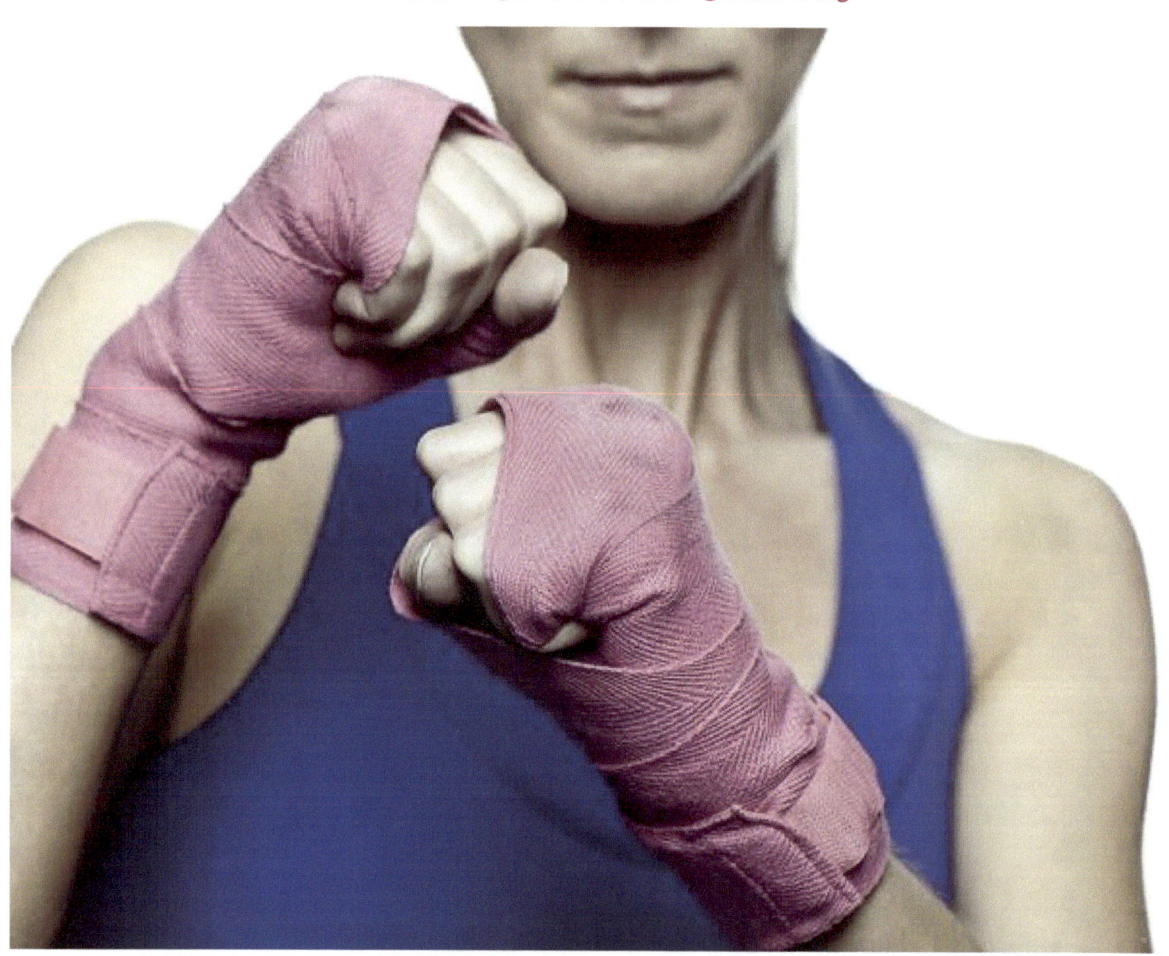

Natural Cancer Treatment by Arlin J. Brown

Arlin J. Brown
Director, The Arlin J. Brown Information Center, Inc.
P.O. Box 251
Fort Belvoir, VA 22060

As an introduction, let me say that for the last ten years I have been the director of a non-profit cancer information center. The purpose of this information center is to gather information on natural, non-toxic and effective treatments for cancer and to disseminating the most valuable information to cancer patients, doctors, researchers and health-minded people. The primary method of disseminating this information is through a book which I have written, entitled March of Truth on Cancer, now in its seventh edition. The book describes 80 safe and valuable cancer treatments which have saved many lives.

In treating cancer successfully, three things must be accomplished:
1. The body must be detoxified.
2. The malignancy must be eliminated, and
3. The body must be regenerated and the deficient nutrients replaced.

While many factors play a role in causing cancer, the primary cause is toxemia. The toxins come from two sources - external and internal. The external poisons come from cooked and refined foods, food additives, preservatives, pesticides, prescription drugs, hormones, etc.

The internal sources of toxins in the body are the waste products of metabolism. Nature intended that these cellular wastes be continually cleansed from the body cells with raw fruits and vegetable, or their juices.

In order to detoxify, one must internally clean out the body. This can be done slowly by changing to a diet of raw fruits and vegetables and their juices - more quickly by also including detoxifying herbs, herb roots, plant roots, sea plants, diatomaceous earth, chlorophyll, vitamins A and E, and high dosages of niacin and Vitamin C. Ginseng helps to detoxify and prevent cancer from forming and metastasizing. Russian ginseng is especially effective. Red ginseng helps to clear out the lymphatic system. Fo-ti-tieng root is a powerful detoxifier. Other good detoxifying herbs include a combination of rhubarb root, golden seal, dandelion root, gota kola, gravel plant, cuscuta arveusis, Irish sea moss, and the enzyme ananase from the pineapple root. Diatomaceous earth tablets eliminate morbid materials in the body. It is rich in silicon, which is Nature's surgeon. The body has many lines of defense against cancer. These include the liver, the pituitary gland, the pancreas, and the thymus. In addition, there are various growth regulators in the body. The detoxification process will cleanse all of the organs. It is very important that the liver and the intestinal tract be cleansed, as well as the pancreas, kidneys, lungs, spleen the endocrine gland, etc. The proper functioning of these organs must be restored.

Remember that there are generally some unpleasant reactions in the body which accompany detoxification, but these are only temporary. These side effects might include nausea, vomiting, weakness, cramps, night sweat, headaches, other aches and pain, nervousness, depression, perhaps palpitation of the heart, and perhaps burning in the rectal area and from the urine because of the acid wastes being eliminated. If the symptoms are too severe and the cancer seems to be breaking up too fast and throwing too much dead toxic material into the bloodstream, then the treatment can be reduced to a more tolerable level, perhaps by reducing the intake of the specific cancer destroyers.

To assist detoxification, a diathermy treatment over the liver, after taking detoxifying herbs, chlorophyll, diatomaceous earth tablets will result in a very good elimination from the liver. Castor oil packs over the liver may also help if the patient is not allergic to it. An American product called Deturge will help to clean the intestinal tract mechanically by forcing black strips of impacted material from the intestines. This product, which swells up in the colon, can be taken before going on the detoxifying herb program.

There are many good organic fruits and vegetables and their freshly made juices which a cancer patient can take. These include grapes, apples, papayas, black cherries, cranberries, beets, carrots, celery, and lactic acid fermented juices and foods. Fruits are best taken in the morning and vegetables in the afternoon and evening. Viscolaticum and fermented muesli are also good. Lactic acid fermented beetroot juice and powder (containing anthracyans) will increase the oxidation in the body cells from 350% to 1,000%. Remember that when wastes and poisons accumulate in the body cells to the point where the cells do not receive sufficient oxygen, the cancer virus becomes active and the cells become malignant. Therefore anything which increases oxidation in the body cells is valuable. One product which puts oxygen directly into the cells after taking it by mouth is Macalozone, an American product which has cured cancer.

The best approach to treating cancer successfully is to use a combination of the best treatments and the best diet, rather than to use a single treatment. One of the most successful treatments now used in the United States is that of Dr. William Kelley of Texas. Dr. Kelley's method includes detoxification, diet, and supplements. This includes two pancreatic enzymes (trypsin and chymotrypsin), vitamins, minerals, blackstrap molasses, raw almonds, a comfrey-pepsin tablet which clears away the excess mucous on the intestinal walls, thereby aiding assimilation, a pre-digested protein product, and a combination of digesting tablets which includes betaine hydrochloric acid, ox bile, papain, pepsin and pancreatin.

The best single treatment for cancer I know of is Tckarina, an injectable derived from seaweed which was developed by Guiseppe Lo Monaco of Tecate, Mexico. It is said to have a cure rate of between 80% and 90% with some 17,000 patients. Among other things, Tekarina acts as a detoxifier and also cures many other ailments besides cancer.

Lactic acid cottage cheese is a good source of protein for the cancer patient. A mixture of cottage cheese and linseed oil is also very good. Personally, I disagree with Dr. Kelley's recommendation of nuts and grains in the early stages of treatment and his use of Epsom salts. Needless to say, the cancer patient should refrain from eating refined and processed foods, toxic cooked foods, meats and anything with harmful additives or which would increase the level of toxins in the body. Correct food combinations should also be followed. Volcanic earth minerals are good for replacing the deficient minerals in the cancer patient. Lactobacillus Bifidus is very important. It should normally comprise about 80% of the intestinal flora, while acidophilus should amount to about 20%. Both should be taken. Incidentally, biopsies are dangerous. For instance, the Squamous cell type of cancer can spread throughout the entire body within 8 minutes after taking a biopsy. There are many other treatments for cancer which I don't have time to discuss now, but you will find many of them in my book, March of Truth on Cancer.

In conclusion, we need to have a better exchange of cancer and health information and also a better exchange of cancer and health products between the United States and Europe. If anyone is interested in exchanging information or in using each other's products, please write to me.

Nobody should die of cancer. Cancer is definitely a curable disease, when safe, non-toxic, effective methods of nature are used.

~ *Speech delivered May 29, 1973 by Arlin J. Brown at the First World Congress on L'Altra Medinia, San Remo, Italy.*

A Plan For Building The Immune System by Lorraine Day, M.D.

Cancer doesn't scare me anymore. I had it . . . and got well with natural, simple therapies that you seldom hear about. I refused mutilating surgery, radiation and chemotherapy because studies in the medical literature and common sense told me that you shouldn't destroy your immune system while you are trying to get well.

The following information is for educational purposes only and should not be construed as prescribing treatment. Treatment should be decided by each individual patient under the advice of a competent health practitioner. However, it is important for individuals to be informed about all options available for treatment and prevention of illness. The underlining basis and documentation for this program of building the immune system are presented in my DVD, "Cancer Doesn't Scare Me Anymore. "

Cancer is a disease of the immune system. Building the immune system is important in combating cancer as well as many other diseases. Disease is not confined to one organ or area but affects the whole body as all parts are interconnected. Therefore, therapy must be a holistic approach to improve all body's systems. A "magic bullet" approach rarely works for any significant illness. The following regimen will help build the immune system for those who are ill or will help prevent disease in those not presently ill.

This is a brief synopsis of the basic three part plan:

1. High quality nutritional intake.

A diet of vegetables, fruit, grains and nuts organically grown without pesticides and prepared to maintain the maximum nutrition outlined in detail in my diodes, including specifics of the Gerson therapy with references provided.

If it can be tolerated by the intestines, at least 50% of the food should be eaten raw, including large quantities of fresh vegetable juices.

Elimination of all processed foods, as well as, salt and sugar (including artificial sweeteners, especially corn syrup).

2. Elimination of toxins from the body by colon cleansing with either enemas, colonics, colon cleansers and/or a high fiber diet.

3. Elimination of toxins from the local environment, including removal of toxic cleaning chemicals from the house and replacement with non-toxic biodegradable cleaners.

Many other specific individual nutritional therapies and supplements, including barley green, Essiac tea and shark cartilage are helpful in certain instances and are presented in some detail in the DVD with numerous resources provided. Many have found that a basic regimen incorporating this three point plan with the addition of specific supplements, depending on the condition, has resulted in major improvements and even elimination of many diseases, including cancer.

In the DVD "Cancer Doesn't Scare Me Anymore" you will learn:

- Why people get cancer. It's not a mystery as some would have you believe.
- How to get well without vomiting and losing your hair.
- Cancer is big business - billions of dollars each year in America alone - and why a cure would hurt Big Business.
- How you can control whether you get sick or stay well and how to avoid buying cancer at the store.

Today, I feel great. Immune building therapy has provided me with maintenance of a full head of hair, excellent energy to continue to work at my regular pace and to walk or run 3 - 5 miles every day, an excellent appetite, freedom from aches and pains, and a positive attitude about my health and life. Over the past few years, I've been bombarded by calls and letters from people wanting to know how I accomplished such a medical feat. Consequently, I recorded my entire story in the DVD I've described above.

The video is available by:

- Visiting www.drday.com/inlex.html#scare
- Calling: 800-574-2437

Why Women in China Don't Get Breast Cancer by Prof. Jane Plant, PhD, CBE

I had no alternative but to die or to try to find a cure for myself. I am a scientist – surely there was a rational explanation for this cruel illness that affects one in 12 women in the UK?

I had suffered the loss of one breast, and undergone radiotherapy. I was now receiving painful chemotherapy, and had been seen by some of the country's most eminent specialists. But, deep down, I felt certain I was facing death. I had a loving husband, a beautiful home and two young children to care for. I desperately wanted to live.

Fortunately, this desire drove me to unearth the facts, some of which were known only to a handful of scientists at the time.

Anyone who has come into contact with breast cancer will know that certain risk factors – such as increasing age, early onset of womanhood, late onset of menopause and a family history of breast cancer – are completely out of our control. But there are many risk factors, which we can control easily.

These "controllable" risk factors readily translate into simple changes that we can all make in our day-to-day lives to help prevent or treat breast cancer. My message is that even advanced breast cancer can be overcome because I have done it.

The first clue to understanding what was promoting my breast cancer came when my husband Peter, who was also a scientist, arrived back from working in China while I was being plugged in for a chemotherapy session.

He had brought with him cards and letters, as well as some amazing herbal suppositories, sent by my friends and science colleagues in China.

The suppositories were sent to me as a cure for breast cancer. Despite the awfulness of the situation, we both had a good belly laugh, and I remember saying that this was the treatment for

breast cancer in China, then, it was little wonder that Chinese women avoided getting the disease. Those words echoed in my mind. Why didn't Chinese women in China get breast cancer? I had collaborated once with Chinese colleagues on a study of links between soil chemistry and disease, and I remembered some of the statistics.

The disease was virtually non-existent throughout the whole country. Only one in 10,000 women in China will die from it, compared to that terrible figure of one in 12 in Britain and the even grimmer average of one in 10 across most Western countries. It is not just a matter of China being a more rural country, with less urban pollution. In highly urbanized Hong Kong, the rate rises to 34 women in every 10,000 but still puts the West to shame. The Japanese cities of Hiroshima and Nagasaki have similar rates. And remember, both cities were attacked with nuclear weapons, so in addition to the usual pollution-related cancers, one would also expect to find some radiation-related cases, too.

The conclusion we can draw from these statistics strikes you with some force. If a Western woman were to move to industrialized, irradiated Hiroshima, she would slash her risk of contracting breast cancer by half. Obviously this is absurd. It seemed obvious to me that some lifestyle factor not related to pollution, urbanization or the environment is seriously increasing the Western woman's chance of contracting breast cancer.

I then discovered that whatever causes the huge differences in breast cancer rates between oriental and Western countries, it isn't genetic.

Scientific research showed that when Chinese or Japanese people move to the West, within one or two generations their rates of breast cancer approach those of their host community.

The same thing happens when oriental people adopt a completely Western lifestyle in Hong Kong. In fact, the slang name for breast cancer in China translates as 'Rich Woman's Disease'. This is because, in China, only the better off can afford to eat what is termed ' Hong Kong food'.

The Chinese describe all Western food, including everything from ice cream and chocolate bars to spaghetti and feta cheese, as "Hong Kong food", because of its availability in the former British colony and its scarcity, in the past, in mainland China.

So it made perfect sense to me that whatever was causing my breast cancer and the shockingly high incidence in this country generally, it was almost certainly something to do with our better-off, middle-class, Western lifestyle. There is an important point for men here, too. I have observed in my research that much of the data about prostate cancer leads to similar conclusions.

According to figures from the World Health Organization, the number of men contracting prostate cancer in rural China is negligible, only 0.5 men in every 100,000. In England, Scotland and Wales, however, this figure is 70 times higher. Like breast cancer, it is a middle-class disease that primarily attacks the wealthier and higher socio-economic groups, those that can afford to eat rich foods.

I remember saying to my husband, "Come on Peter, you have just come back from China. What is it about the Chinese way of life that is so different? Why don't they get breast cancer?"

We decided to utilize our joint scientific backgrounds and approach it logically.

We examined scientific data that pointed us in the general direction of fats in diets. Researchers had discovered in the 1980s that only 14% of calories in the average Chinese diet were from fat, compared to almost 36% in the West. But the diet I had been living on for years before I contracted breast cancer was very low in fat and high in fiber. Besides, I knew as a scientist that fat intake in adults has not been shown to increase risk for breast cancer in most investigations that have followed large groups of women for up to a dozen years.

Then one day something rather special happened. Peter and I have worked together so closely over the years that I am not sure which one of us first said: "The Chinese don't eat dairy produce!"

It is hard to explain to a non-scientist the sudden mental and emotional 'buzz' you get when you know you have had an important insight. It's as if you have had a lot of pieces of a jigsaw in your mind, and suddenly, in a few seconds, they all fall into place and the whole picture is clear.

Suddenly I recalled how many Chinese people were physically unable to tolerate milk, how the Chinese people I had worked with had always said that milk was only for babies, and how one of my close friends, who is of Chinese origin, always politely turned down the cheese course at dinner parties.

I knew of no Chinese people who lived a traditional Chinese life who ever used cow or other dairy food to feed their babies. The tradition was to use a wet nurse but never, ever, dairy products.

Culturally, the Chinese find our Western preoccupation with milk and milk products very strange. I remember entertaining a large delegation of Chinese scientists shortly after the ending of the Cultural Revolution in the 1980s.

On advice from the Foreign Office, we had asked the caterer to provide a pudding that contained a lot of ice cream. After inquiring what the pudding consisted of, all of the Chinese, including their interpreter, politely but firmly refused to eat it, and they could not be persuaded to change their minds.

At the time we were all delighted and ate extra portions!

Milk, I discovered, is one of the most common causes of food allergy. Over 70% of the world's population is unable to digest the milk sugar, lactose, which has led nutritionists to believe that this is the normal condition for adults, not some sort of deficiency. Perhaps nature is trying to tell us that we are eating the wrong food.

Before I had breast cancer for the first time, I had eaten a lot of dairy produce, such as skimmed milk, low-fat cheese and yoghurt. I had used it as my main source of protein. I also ate cheap but lean minced beef, which I now realized was probably often ground-up dairy cow.

In order to cope with the chemotherapy I received for my fifth case of cancer, I had been eating organic yoghurts as a way of helping my digestive tract to recover and repopulate my gut with 'good' bacteria.

Recently, I discovered that way back in 1989 yoghurt had been implicated in ovarian cancer. Dr Daniel Cramer of Harvard University studied hundreds of women with ovarian cancer, and had them record in detail what they normally ate. Wish I'd been made aware of his findings when he had first discovered them.

Following Peter's and my insight into the Chinese diet, I decided to give up not just yoghurt but all dairy produce immediately. Cheese, butter, milk and even many proprietary brands of margarine marketed as soya, sunflower or olive oil, spreads, yoghurt and anything else that contained dairy produce - it went down the sink or in the rubbish.

It is surprising how many products, including commercial soups, biscuits and cakes, contain some form of dairy produce. I therefore became an avid reader of the small print on food labels.

Up to this point, I had been steadfastly measuring the progress of my fifth cancerous lump with calipers and plotting the results. Despite all the encouraging comments and positive feedback from my doctors and nurses, my own precise observations told me the bitter truth.

My first chemotherapy sessions had produced no effect – the lump was still the same size.

Then I eliminated dairy products. Within days, the lump started to shrink. About two weeks after my second chemotherapy session and one week after giving up dairy produce, the lump in my neck started to itch. Then it began to soften and to reduce in size. The line on the graph, which had shown no change, was now pointing downwards as the tumor got smaller and smaller.

And, very significantly, I noted that instead of declining exponentially (a graceful curve) as cancer is meant to do, the tumor's decrease in size was plotted on a straight line heading off the bottom of the graph, indicating a cure, not suppression (or remission) of the tumor.

One Saturday afternoon after about six weeks of excluding all dairy produce from my diet, I practiced an hour of meditation then felt for what was left of the lump. I couldn't find it. Yet I was very experienced at detecting cancerous lumps – I had discovered all five cancers on my own.

I went downstairs and asked my husband to feel my neck. He could not find any trace of the lump either.

On the following Thursday I was due to be seen by my cancer specialist at Charing Cross Hospital in London. He examined me thoroughly, especially my neck where the tumor had been. He was initially bemused and then delighted as he said, "I cannot find it."
None of my doctors, it appeared, had expected someone with my type and stage of cancer (which had clearly spread to the lymph system) to survive, let alone be so hale and hearty.

My specialist was as overjoyed as I was. When I first discussed my ideas with him he was understandably skeptical. But I understand that he now uses maps showing cancer mortality in China in his lectures, and recommends a non-dairy diet to his cancer patients.

I now believe that the link between dairy produce and breast cancer is similar to the link between smoking and lung cancer. I believe that identifying the link between breast cancer and dairy +produce, and then developing a diet specifically targeted at maintaining the health of my breast and hormone system, cured me.

It was difficult for me, as it may be for you, to accept that a substance as 'natural' as milk might have such ominous health implications. But I am a living proof that it works and, starting from tomorrow, I shall reveal the secrets of my revolutionary action plan.

Laetrile: Cancer Cure or Quackery? by Del Schrader

The battle over Laetrile as a cancer treatment medication has been furiously waged in the media, in the courts, in laboratories, on street corners and in studio sessions. A dead woman was involved as a plaintiff in a suit filed in San Jose. It contends that the State Department of Health's 1963 order banning the use of Laetrile in cancer treatment is unconstitutional. Josephine Bergman of Altos, listed as a plaintiff, died after being ill with cancer for over a year. She was 48 and a patient of Dr. Stewart M. Jones of Palo Alto. The suit said Stanford Hospital refused to allow Dr. Jones to prescribe and administer Laetrile to Mrs. Bergman. Laetrile, also known as Vitamin B-17, is a substance made from apricot and peach pits. Oddly enough, although banned as a cancer treatment, controversial Laetrile may be used as a nutritional supplement.

Mrs. Betty Lee Morales, a Los Angeles nutritional consultant, told the Herald Examiner, "Cancer is the only disease controlled politically. A doctor can put ice cream on an arthritic knee, but can only use surgery, radiation or chemotherapy in the treatment of cancer, otherwise, he can be put in jail. More than 20 foreign nations now use Laetrile, but the American Medical Association (AMA) and the Food and Drug Administration (FDA) keep it a crime in the U.S." Mrs. Morales counters, "The biggest problem the U.S. faces is solving the cancer problem, but it's tough getting information to the people. Why, I have watched one of the biggest daily newspapers and one of the biggest TV networks buckle under the establishments." Mrs. Lorraine Rosenthal, cofounder with Mrs. Morales of the Cancer Control Society in Hollywood, told the Herald Examiner, "They say Laetrile pills are being peddled on the streets of Tijuana, but Californians don't have to go to Mexico for Laetrile. They can buy it here in California under the name of Amygdalin from four or five sources. Remember, Laetrile is only a phone call away. But for those patients who go to Mexico, a medical doctor, Ernesto Contreras, treats many cancer patients in his office in Playa de Tijuana.

Millions of words have gone into the Great Laetrile Debate. Dean Burk of the National Cancer Institute, recently stated, "I don't know whether Laetrile is any good, or how good it is - but l believe it should be tested so we can find out. So far, all the actions of the FDA have been based on prejudice, ignorance and fraud." Dr. Burk cited several Laetrile tests around the world since the father-son team of Dr. Ernst Krebs Jr. and Sr. in 1950 discovered the biochemical abilities of apricot kernels in San Francisco.

The tests:

- Sloan-Kettering, where mice bearing spontaneous mammary cancer were treated with amounts from one to two grams of Laetrile per kilogram of body weight. The results showed spread of cancer inhibited, with the animals showing greater health.

- Scind laboratories, University of San Francisco, where 400 test rats bore 256 carcinoma. Two hundred rats treated with B-17 showed an 80% increase in life span over those not treated with B-17.

- Pasteur Institute, Paris, where researchers maintained a human cancer strain in mice, their life span was increased and tumor growth delayed up to an amazing 100% by use of B-17, Dr. Burk's figures revealed. Institute Von Ardenne, Dresden, Germany, obtained similar findings.

But the battle to control the minds of men and women continues. The Cancer Control Journal had a picture of comedian Red Buttons and his wife on page one with the caption: Red Buttons says, "Laetrile saved my wife from death by cancer."

A final word from Betty Morales: "The trouble with Laetrile is that more than 90% of all patients have already gone through chemo-therapy, radiation or surgery, but the late Dr. Ernst T. Krebs Sr. still cured 98% of those who came to him. He cured more than 1,000 before he died at 94. I'm proud of the 10 years I spent with him." For Laetrile sources do a web search for "Laetrile".

Wheat Grass and Laetrile Credited for Beating Cancer by Louis L. Wahal

It was in May of 1977, that I found out that I was suffering from a deadly, inoperable and incurable form of cancer, called Grade 4 Un-differential Neoplasm. My eye was sticking out of the socket. I had two lumps on my forehead and another lump as big as a golf ball a little to the side and right under my chin. It was like the roots of a tree spreading through my sinuses and all thorough my head. I had just one thing in my favor. The cancer had not yet reached my brain. It was a very fast growing cancer. You could almost see it grow. After trying everything that medical science could do for me, I was told to go home and get my house in order and to get ready to die. This came from Mayo Clinic in Rochester, MN. They said there was nothing more they could do for me.

It was at this point that my eldest son, David, said, "Dad, why don't you try Mexico?" We didn't have much faith in them at this time but we had run out of alternatives and felt that we had nothing to lose. So without further ado, my wife and I were off to Mexico. It was there that I underwent treatment with large doses of Laetrile, vitamins, and enzymes prescribed by Dr. Contreras at the Centro Medico Del Mar Clinic Tijuana. I had taken a series of radiation treatments at the Mayo Clinic prior to this and I was advised by Dr. Contreras to go back and complete the series of treatments. Dr. Contreras wasn't too hopeful about my recovery either but he said that he would try. I had 44 cobalt treatments in all.

We had finished the last session of treatments at Rochester and my wife and I were ready to go home. We had some time to spare so we went to a local Health Food Store in Rochester just to browse around and get acquainted with some of the new foods we were going to become familiar with. It was then that we spotted a bottle of green grass pills. Virginia, my wife, had been doing some reading about this new kind of health care using foods instead of drugs, and we had been told in Mexico that I should have Wheat Grass. We were unable to grow it because we were on the run all the time, going to doctors and hospitals. "Could this be the answer we were looking for?" my wife said, we had spent all of our pocket money so we didn't have enough money to buy the bottle of green pills. We went home without them. Virginia was restless. She just couldn't calm down. We had been doing a great deal of praying, and it was at this point that something moved her to go to the phone and call the store in Rochester. She asked to have 2 bottles shipped to us C.O.D. The pills arrived a couple of days later and I began taking them at once. We had no one to direct us on how to take them or even how many, but the directions on the label said to take 12 to 14 a day, so that was what I did.

Within three days, the lumps began to get softer and my skin began to get pink again. You readers can't believe the amount of ecstasy and new strength that went through our hearts and minds. I kept taking the pills every day. We were so thankful that we prayed on our hands and knees telling God that we were going to do everything in our power to tell the world that they don't have to die from cancer. Within three weeks my face looked normal again. Of course I was not yet well. I had lost a lot of weight and I had a lot of recovering to do from all the damage that the cobalt treatments had done.

To this day, now four years later I have not had a single setback. I now take better care of myself, making sure that I get plenty of rest and, although at first I was on a very strict and nutritious diet, I now add a few more pleasurable things to my diet. I still stay away from sugars, salt, red meat (I do a little beef once in a great while), I eat whole grain breads, and plenty of fresh fruits and vegetables,. My wife and I have been living a completely normal life. Last spring in April, we enjoyed a five week trip to Hawaii and Australia. We both enjoy travel very much. I have for over a year now been able to cut my Laetrile intake down to only one tablet a day. I really don't think I still need it but I don't want to take any chances since things are going so good. I still take my 14 green pills faithfully every day.

I thank God every day for this great gift of life, for giving me the healing and leading me to these green Wheat Grass pills.

Conclusion

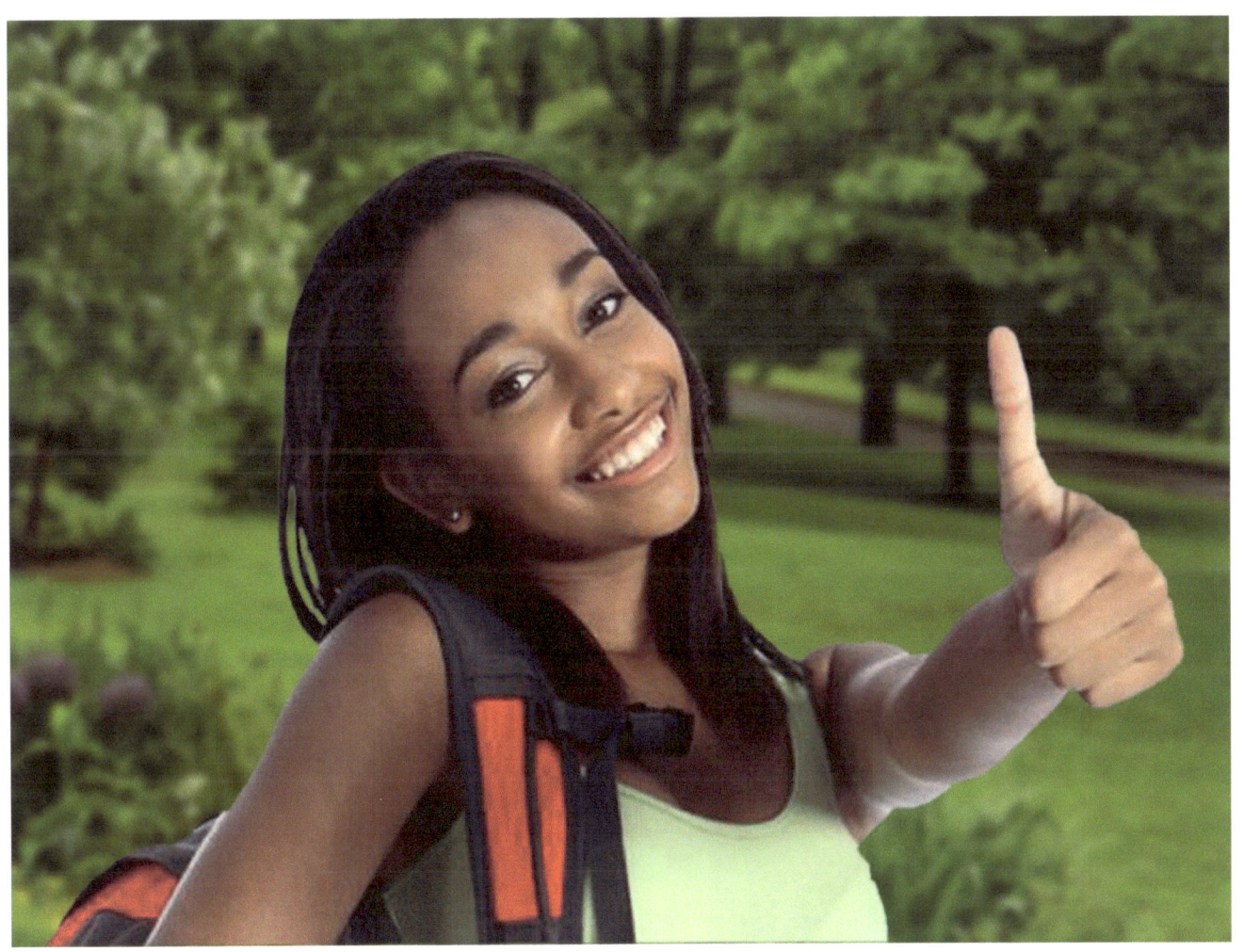

When people are asked why they choose alternative therapy, one common reason they give is that the treatments are consistent with their views of health and wellness. Something everyone should consider when choosing a treatment is- what does health mean to you, what areas of your life do you feel most healthy and what areas do you think you need to work on and improve?

I hope that this book has given you enough approaches to consider. And remember, it's imperative that you choose a path that feels right for you. This path includes the right therapy, the right level of commitment from you (and maybe your family) and most importantly, the right practitioner to help you through your journey to health and wellness.

Also, please remember that your needs may change over time. What you needed a few months ago, may not be what you need today. Every once in a while, you may wish to look over the therapies you are using and assess how well they are working for you. If you are looking for different results, you may need to choose a different form of treatment. I've given you **190** different methods to try out, so you won't be short of ideas!

In the end, I hope that you have found this book helpful and the info and methods in it as beneficial to you as they have been to many cancer survivors. I would love to hear your own survival stories. Please feel free to contact me with any questions, comments or stories at Sage@SageCrystal.net. I would love to hear from you about how helpful you have found the information in the book to be! Good luck on your journey to wellness and freedom from cancer with alternative methods! For additional resources, visit:

Sage Crystal

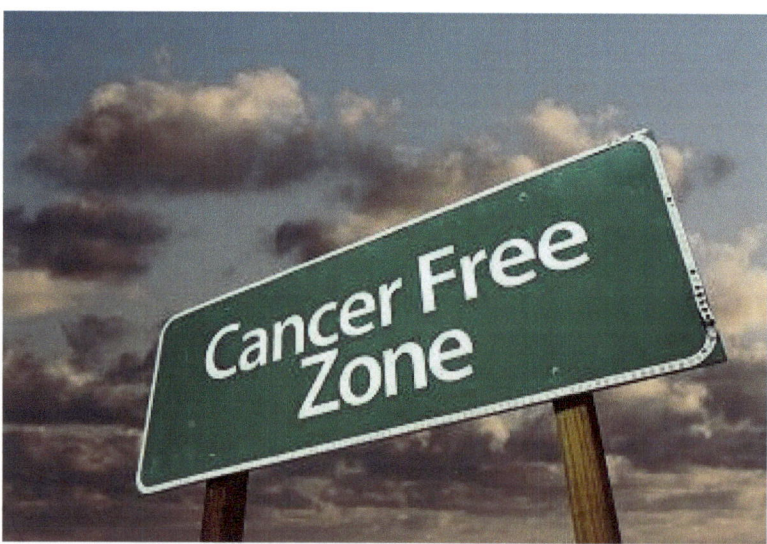